The Sexy Bitch's Book
of
Doing It,
Getting It
and
Giving It

The Sexy Bitch's Book of Doing It, Getting It and Giving It

FLIC EVERETT

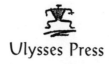

Ulysses Press

Published in the United States by
Ulysses Press
P.O. Box 3440
Berkeley, CA 94703
www.ulyssespress.com

ISBN 1-56975-391-1
Library of Congress Control Number: 2003109422

First published in Great Britain in 2002 by Channel 4 Books,
an imprint of Pan Macmillan Ltd.

Printed in Canada by Transcontinental Printing

1 3 5 7 9 8 6 4 2

Cover artwork: Getty Images/Thinkstock
Cover design: Sarah Levin

Distributed in the U.S.A. by Publishers Group West

Flic Everett would like to thank Lou Paget and Anne Hooper.

contents

introduction

Sex can be the greatest event in the world. But it can also be less fun than turning up to the circus a week late, finding only a patch of flattened grass where you were expecting a three-ring extravaganza. There's so much written, spoken and discussed when it comes to sex, you'd think we'd all be sexperts, tweaking nipples in our sleep, bringing partners to dizzying orgasm with one hand while polishing our tool-kit of vibrators with the other.

The truth is, though, sex is never that simple—how much you enjoy it depends on a number of factors, from whom you're doing it with, to how tired you are, to whether the bed squeaks, to how you're feeling about yourself.

Sometimes we want a ten-course banquet of physical delights, other times sexual fast food is all we crave. Real sex is funny, enjoyable, and occasionally silly, and when you're with the right person, it can include everything from a reassuring cuddle to an epic journey of discovery.

Far too much sex advice is aimed at people who don't appear to be having a real sex life at all—they're simply mating on some strange planet where emotions don't count and everyone's a master of yoga. *The Sexy Bitch's Book of Doing It, Getting It and Giving It*, however, is all about real people who enjoy real sex.

What real people having real sex need most are a few pointers that make sure all types of sex are as enjoyable as they possibly can be. All the tips in *The Sexy Bitch's Book of Doing It, Getting It and Giving It* have been tried and tested by real couples. Experts who truly know what they're talking about help out, too, and not one of them suggests that swinging naked from a chandelier is a valid or even erotic way to pass the time.

So if you want to feel inadequate, confused, and worried that your sex life is hopelessly dull and useless, go buy another sex manual. If, however, you want a lot of practical tips, clear explanations, and enjoyable experiences ... then read on.

But before you do, keep this in mind: Your sexual health is your responsibility and safe sex should be your priority at all times. "Safe" sex, using condoms, dental dams and other prophylactics, is no less erotic, and it's certainly more fun than dealing with an STD or unplanned pregnancy. OK. Now on to the juicy bits....

1 foreplay

If there's anyone who doesn't know by now that foreplay is generally necessary for good sex, they've almost certainly been living in some Jurassic swamp practicing their hot moves on the last remaining diplodocus. Having said that, while most men and women are eager enough to rev up their partners with some hand and tongue action, plenty of them are still a little unsure and approach the whole thing as if they're constructing some origami swan, complete with flaps and bits that won't stick down. Foreplay is, simply, the art of turning your partner on enough to make them want to have sex—though it can be enjoyable as an experience in its own right.

For men, that might be simply a case of "Want to fuck?," though even the most hair-trigger man will still appreciate having his penis handled delicately first. And for women, it's a far lengthier process, involving chat, jokes, stroking, cuddling, licking, nibbling and squeezing. Unless, of course, she's already desperate for it—and even then, you need to devote a good half-hour to her bodily needs first.

Foreplay begins, as they say, "outside the bedroom." We're not going to bother with all the "it begins with a mental connection" stuff, though, because the assumption is that if you're about to get naked you already have some kind of connection going on, even if it's only like two faulty electric wires twisted together.

Foreplay isn't just about manipulating each other's genitals to an explosive point of no return, it's about touching, stroking and caressing each other before you even head below the waistline. Women's bodies are programmed to respond to the softest, most featherlike of touches, and sometimes the merest brush of lips on neck can result in feelings of orgasmic intensity. Men can be a little more claylike in their responses, and may need a firmer hand applied to their erogenous zones. But that doesn't mean they can't appreciate gentle caresses or being softly stroked. It is possible to get in the mood for sex before you even see each other though—by talking dirty.

talking dirty

Foreplay isn't just about physical frolicking—it's about getting into the mood for sex, and for some men that means a quick scrub with soap on a rope and a brief thought about Sarah Michelle Gellar in a corset. For women it's a little more complex than that. This is where talking dirty comes in. Given that sex is at least as much mental stimulation as physical—well, good sex is—it pays to rev up the engine before attempting to drive the car. So "nice tits, get your pants off"

TIP

An easy way to get into talking dirty if you find it a little difficult at first is to use words normally associated with food ("boil me now ... put me on a slow roast and turn me halfway through"—no, I'm joking). Words like eat, lick, suck, taste, and nibble are useful. And using blunt words for acts is better than the medical terms—"vagina" sounds like you're a doctor about to perform an examination, whereas "cunt" is suitably earthy and basic.

Dirty talk doesn't have to be very articulate. If the problem is that you worry you'll lose the thread halfway through, don't—he really won't care. Even a few phrases thrown in here and there will do the job—"fuck me hard" doesn't require any great mental powers. To begin with, get three dice, and write six adjectives on one—such as "hot," "sexy," "wet" and so on. Then on the second, write six verbs—"fuck," "touch," "thrust"—and on the final one, write six nouns. Then throw the dice, and all you need to come up with are the joining-up words—and say them out loud.

probably won't do it, but a little more sophisticated dirty talk just might.

You can e-mail your partner during the day, and state a few things you might like to do to him later—but it helps if he's between meetings, not actually in one. Typing "I want your hot cock inside me," just as the boss is standing behind him waiting for him to download the quarterly figures, is not sexy, it's just stupid. But once you're sure he's free to communicate, go right ahead and be as rude as possible.

Text messages are an equally sexy way of getting your message across—though make sure you don't become such an expert at teen-style text language that he has absolutely no idea what you're talking about. A quick "I want u 2 cum on my tits," however, should leave him in no doubt about your intentions. And hopefully, his colleague hasn't borrowed his phone for the afternoon.

Phone sex is another way of getting yourselves hot, by talking each other to the point of orgasm—"now I'm touching your hard cock … now I'm sliding my hand up and down it …" style of chit-chat

> **TIP**
>
> Because men are so visual, if you are going to e-mail or text him with wild promises of things you're going to do to him, explain it so he gets the picture. Instead of saying "have surprise 4 u later," say "will give u blow job on way home frm wrk," for example. Though if your journey home involves a packed commuter train, maybe that isn't the time …. Equally, when he e-mails you he shouldn't make demands, he should simply outline what he'd like to do to you. Of course, he may well get a blow job, but telling you he'll go down on you for hours will be a more appealing text message, right?

should work. Of course, he has to reciprocate, and tell you how much he wants to be inside your beautiful cunt, fucking you senseless …. With talking dirty, never forget, however, that it's only a short step from "huge turn-on" to "sounding stupid." Anything that veers too much toward porn-star small talk is never going to work. So "ride my tool, bitch" will simply sound silly, as will "fill my tunnel with your hot cum"—unless it happens to work for you, in which case go ahead, and good luck with finding a distributor.

Find a language that is intimate and sexual for you, whether that's "Poppa's baby rabbit wants his big carrot" or simply "I want you in me, right now." If you're too shy for dirty foreplay-talk, then texting and e-mailing are godsends. Don't ignore their potential.

little kisses

Obviously, kissing is an element of foreplay. But most of us mastered the basic make-out maneuver by the second year of high school, so we'll assume you know pretty much what you should be doing with your tongue by now, at least when it happens to be in someone else's mouth. When it comes to foreplay, it's what to do with it when it's anywhere else on his body that matters.

And while most sex manuals suggest you should "lick him all over," that's just going to make him feel like a giant kitten. That may work for your guy, but for the average guy, a full lick-bath will just leave him feeling like he should be scratching for fleas and chasing a mouse. The tongue should be used sparingly, but effectively—like garlic in pasta dishes. A little can make all the difference, but, for some, too much may be just darn right unpleasant.

Start with a delicate trail along the side of his neck, just below his ear—you may want to swirl it into the hollow crevice of his shoulder-blade too, which will activate a whole bunch of tiny nerves. Alternate this with tiny, brushing kisses—few guys want their shoulder kissed, but there's a big difference between that and light stimulation of the skin. The back of his neck is another hotspot, which will respond with

---

TIP

Shaving your pubes can be a thrill for both of you—shaving his will immediately make his penis look bigger, while shaving yours is sexy because it exposes more of your labia. It also means that when you have sex there's more friction, and your clitoris gets more effectively ground into. Shaving, however, is incredibly itchy when it grows back; waxing is a more attractive option—and also makes it easier to trim neatly, particularly if your hair tends to be bushy. If shaving is a turn-on for you, then shave each other—but only when you're sober, alright?

great alacrity to a little tongue-flicking, particularly if you move down to the top of his spine and swirl the tip (of your tongue, not his spine, silly) in small circles.

Most men don't like having their faces licked—back to kittens—but a little kissing and licking of the nipples is a very fine thing. Learn from men's mistakes, and don't twiddle them like you're tuning into an alternative radio station. A light swish of the tongue, back and forth, across them, or a little gentle sucking should be enough to fire up the connection to his penis almost instantly. If he isn't in touch with the Power of Nipple, he's probably got all sorts of hang-ups about it being "womanly" or something, so it's your job to put him straight, and explain that god gave men nipples for a reason, and it clearly wasn't to feed babies.

If you're inclined, you can kiss and lick his feet, but I personally can think of about fifty things to do that might be more fun, starting with "make a papier maché model of Hong Kong" and ending with "arrange a series of roly polies in order of size." Still, if it works for

TIP

If you're going to take control in bed and initiate sex, you have to be able to state what you want. A men's magazine survey found that the most common response from women when asked what they want from their partners is "I don't care," or "whatever you feel like." Of course you care! You're just too shy to tell him so. Practice by saying "that feels great" or "mmm, that's lovely," then when he asks you can at least say, "I loved that thing you were doing when I said it felt amazing." Otherwise you'll both be left unsatisfied—so pick up on his cues, too.

He doesn't necessarily understand that kissing doesn't have to lead to sex. To a man's brain, if you're getting hot and heavy and kissing, you're basically saying, "I want to have sex with you, right now." To yours, you may just be saying, "I really like you, and I really feel like kissing." So make it clear—just murmur, "I love making out with no other expectations sometimes, it's so sexy." That should do it.

you, you go girlfriend and suck those toes. Of course, if you expect him to suck yours, you may have to reciprocate, though you may wish to point out that your feet are probably quite fragrant and your toenails are painted a lovely pink shade, unlike the scaly yellow monstrosities that are most men's extremities.

So restrain your licking and nibbly kissing to his inner thighs. The worst thing about them should be the hairs that get caught in your teeth. Aside from that, inner thighs are a source of great wonder and delight—they are packed with nerve endings, just waiting to be stimulated, with a direct connection to the genitalia. Just lick and kiss your way up them, stopping just short of the boxer-short line (whether he's wearing them or not) to have him writhing with desire. This works just as well, if not better, for you too, of course—he should use his hand to stroke one thigh while kissing and trailing his tongue up the inside of the other. Butts respond to kissing beautifully, too— we're not talking about the inner workings at this point, that's a whole other chapter—the cheeks themselves only require the lightest touch to spring into life. Kiss the hollow at the bottom of the back, and run your tongue in circles over his butt—unless it's spotty, in

Using little brushes on each other's skin feels like being touched all over by delicate fingertips—and therefore, great. Get a little selection of artists' paintbrushes, feather dusters, ostrich feathers and the like, and try them out on each other's skin, moving from fairly hard bristles (no, not a scrubbing brush) down to the tip of a feather to see what works best. There are so many nerves in the skin that just being touched with a soft brush can be a deeply erotic experience.

which case you are officially exempt from all butt-related duties. He should kiss yours too, and can even try the odd, gentle, bite—we're not talking about him sinking his teeth in like it's a club sandwich, though.

If you want to, you can try the full kiss and lick experience on each other's hands, but it might be a bit too similar to a whole knights-about-to-joust scenario, as he kisses your hand and licks your wrist. Be sure to try the ears—perhaps the part of the body that responds most effectively to kissing and nibbling. Be very careful, however, to do this quietly, or it'll sound like someone eating chips in your ear canal.

If you're short on time, though, have a lot of kissing and licking to deposit, and aren't sure where to head for, then go straight to the erogenous zones without passing "Go." They are butt, breasts (or nipples for men, obviously), neck and lips. Some individuals may have urgently erotic elbows, but it's rare—so stick with what you know. And never lick like a mommy cat trying to dislodge a lingering flea.

massage

If licking all over sounds like a whole lot of effort, then offer a massage instead. Massages are not just for sports stars and men at sex clubs. It is, in fact, the perfect way to turn each other on, relax muscles that are knotted more tightly than oak tree roots, and get as close as you can to orgasm without actually having one. A really good massage should leave your whole body feeling flooded with sensual delight, with all your dormant nerve-endings waking up like Rip Van Winkle after a hundred-year nap. You can choose just to massage a small area—shoulders, butt, penis—or go for the full-body meltdown-massage, which should take at least an hour if you're doing it right. A few brisk jiggles of the shoulders does not count as doing it right, incidentally.

how to give a sexy massage

He (or you) should lie on his front—that way you're not going to be distracted by his bobbing erection every time you glance down. Cover your hands in scented massage oil and then warm them. Begin at the neck, by placing your hands on either side and stroking lightly upward just under his ears. Then move your thumbs down to the top of his spine and rub in small circles, without pressing too hard—remember, you aren't dealing with sporting injuries, merely trying to activate erotic rushes of feeling. Move right down his spine, pressing and molding with your thumbs, and when you reach the bottom, sweep your hands across his butt cheeks. Never taking your hands off his skin, sweep your palms back up again, then work your thumbs just under his shoulder blades to gently push away tension. Once you've dealt with any basic knots, you can get flirtier—if you have long nails, scrape them (lightly, we're not onto S&M yet) across his back and run them down his spine, or use them to stroke patterns on his skin. If not, just use your fingertips to caress the sides of his body—a horribly neglected area—and trail along his spine. If you really want to give him a sensual massage, finish off by covering your breasts in oil and lying on his back, rubbing yourself up and down. Of course, he'll want to turn over immediately and have sex with you, but don't let him—it's all about arousing him slowly.

If you're dying for a turn yourself, stop at this point—but if you're going for the full effect, now's the time to give his butt a good kneading. Just take a cheek in each hand, and squeeze and release as if you're making a particularly tasty loaf, then work your way down to the tops of his thighs, where you turn your fingers inward, and continue to massage his inner thighs, going as close as you dare—gently—to his balls. Work up and down, and if you want to you can move onto his calves, but if so, be aware that a calf massage is a little too physical therapist-friendly to be truly erotic. A foot massage can be arousing,

TIP

When you're giving a massage, you should both be naked. It's no fun if only one of you is playing. Straddle his butt, leaning on your hands so your weight is mainly on your upper back, and use it as leverage to place the pressure of your hands on his shoulder blades. The back massage feels nice, but the thing that really matters is whether parts of you are grinding into his butt as you massage. If so, his muscular tensions will be dissipated in a matter of minutes, I'm sure—particularly if you then suggest a full frontal massage, and adopt the same straddling position for this one, too.

When he's massaging you, allow him to give you a genital massage. This isn't simply a matter of placing his hand over your genitals and rubbing away—though that can be nice. A correct labial massage involves a technique known as "wibbling"—sounds stupid, feels great. He should use his fingers to gently pull and release all the way up and down each side of the labia. I said "gently." He can go as far as the clitoris, then go back down the other side, without removing his hands at all—and without actually touching your clit—to drive you wild with anticipation.

too, but for many, feet are the work of the devil, and best avoided, however attractive the legs attached to them may be. If you don't fear feet, though, use the ball of your thumb to rub gently around the edge of the foot, and work your way into the middle, pressing lightly. According to reflexologists, each part corresponds to a different part of the body, so if your partner suddenly gets a terrible pain in his liver, you're probably being too rough. Firm enough not to tickle, not so firm that he's in agony is the basic rule of massage—and that counts for everywhere.

Of course, you can massage the genitals, too—but even touching them is a whole new, er, ballgame, and instantly moves your massage from "innocently pleasurable" to "downright thrilling."

touching breasts

Touching breasts is simple. Just treat them gently, never pull, poke, tug or jiggle them—they are not beanbags handed out to kindergarten children, they are sensitive organs in their own right that must be treated with respect. Respectful treatment can include stroking the whole breast area, caressing it with the fingertips, gradually drawing closer to the nipple, which will be rubbed between thumb and forefinger, or lightly tweaked, or stroked. It should not, however, be twiddled, flicked, pulled or pressed, because try as he might, he will never get Jazz FM on your breasts.

The tongue is a very useful addition to breast-fondling—he should use it to lick delicately across your breasts and shoulders, and finally activate your nipples by flicking it across them, or circling it on them. Nipples can be sucked, gently—if he does it too hard, all sorts of comedic noises might ensue—and they can also be licked very successfully. Breasts are simple—think gentle and he can't go too badly wrong.

touching the parts

This is where it starts to get complicated. Because the genitals are a mass of nerve-endings more tangled and complex than an electricity substation, if you're going to stimulate them, it has to be done correctly, or you will simply cause pain and annoyance. Many a guy has

---

TIP

It seems obvious as sex tips go—but that doesn't make it less valid. A huge number of grown women have no idea what their genitals look like. So in order to get a good look and stand any chance of finding the relevant areas when you're masturbating, it's a very good idea to get a hand mirror and a decent light, and have a look. Once you know where your clitoris and vagina are and what they look like, it's much easier to touch yourself in a way that works—and to teach him to do the same.

TIP

A handy way to get yourself in the mood for sex quickly and easily is to focus on a sexy memory. Close your eyes and fully experience it again—how it felt, what you thought at the time, what it looked like … often the day after an intense sexual experience, you're raring to go again because the memory is so fresh, you're still turned on. By reconnecting with that memory, you'll feel that wave of lust all over again—and hey, so what if it was with an ex-boyfriend? It's not like you need to tell him what you're thinking about, is it?

assumed his girlfriend's writhing in ecstasy when she is, in fact, simply attempting to get away from his ham-fisted attempts at getting her off. It shouldn't be that difficult but, in truth, sadly, it is. Even the penis, which many women assume is an idiot-proof device, can be handled wrongly. Treating each other's genitals like baby toys—pulling, prodding, violent jiggling and the like—is a profoundly bad idea. Think of yourself as Aladdin holding the magic lamp—you have to rub in exactly the right way to unleash the orgasm-genie. Though if he's wearing underwear that actually say "rub gently and a genie will appear" on the front, you don't have to do anything except catch the next plane out of town.

handling her parts

Make him memorize this section so well that he can recite it backward on demand. Because only then can you be sure that he actually knows what he's doing. For men, the old "what's a clitoris?" dark ages are largely over, but just because they know what one is and where it is—

well, most do, but for those who missed out on remedial biology class, it's the little tiny pea-shaped thing tucked inside her labia, at the point where her legs join together—doesn't mean that they know what to do with it. Some believe a steady, grinding pressure is required. Others flick it around like it's a pinball flipper. Still others approach it like a dangerous insect, giving it a little tap, then retreating in terror. All of these methods are basically hopeless. Never mind whether she orgasms or not, she's not even going to get to the first level of enjoyment with this kind of action.

The first rule of clitoral stimulation is lubrication. To put it bluntly, he's never going to get anywhere attempting to rub a dry clitoris. If she isn't wet enough—and women only get wet when they're thoroughly turned on—then he has to use an artificial lubricant such as KY Jelly. This has the effect of allowing his fingers to slide back and forth without any painful friction—and tragically, many men are still unaware that their attempts at clitoris-based passion are simply agonizing because they didn't make sure it was wet enough before they galloped in with their rough fingers. The clitoris is the single most

TIP

Men should never use the "dip test" to check whether you're wet enough to have sex—you know, the one where he twiddles your nipples, kisses you a bit, then thrusts his hand into your underwear and prods his finger in the direction of your vagina, to see if you're even slightly lubricated. It's not a terribly classy way to find out—so if he is venturing down there, it's polite to stay and actually stimulate your clitoris. That way, you almost certainly will be ready by the time he wants to go any further.

Women tend to be much more inhibited about their bodies than men are, and consequently they find it harder to let go and enjoy sex, because they're worrying what their butt looks like, or thinking their stomach's hanging down. Two things—build up your own confidence by dimming the lights, lighting candles, wearing your sexiest clothes or underwear, and more importantly, try to accept that he really does want you and he really isn't looking at your stretch marks. Because he's just glad to be there.

sensitive part of a woman (if you discount her feelings regarding the size of her ass) and must be treated as if you're buffing up a precious jewel, rather than the army boot-polishing antics that many men favor. So before you do anything else, lubricate—a pea-sized amount is enough. If you have no KY to hand, saliva is better than nothing, but try not to make hacking noises like a 13-year-old boy at a bus stop. Just lick your finger, OK?

Once you've located the clitoris, make small circles around it with your fingertip, or two fingertips. You'll be able to tell if you're doing it right because she will make noises of appreciation. If you're doing it wrong, she'll catch her breath and bite her lip and look pained. How hard can it be to tell? You can either go straight for her orgasm, without passing go, by maintaining a steady rhythm, building up the speed slightly as she starts to gasp, or you can take the scenic bus route, and begin by stroking her pubic hair, then stroke her outer labia, before pressing more firmly and reaching her inner parts— you can circle your finger around her vagina, and push it in a little way, remembering that only the first 3 inches have nerve-endings.

TIP

Saliva is a very useful lubricant, but only in the absence of anything else. If you can, buy a manufactured one such as KY Jelly or Astroglide (mmm!) because they're properly formulated to replicate vaginal lubrication and feel much nicer—plus they don't immediately dry, which saliva does. Even if you have no trouble producing your own lubrication, it helps to have some for hand jobs, or very lengthy sex sessions—and make sure it's water-based, as oil-based products can damage condoms.

You're unlikely to reach the G-spot with your finger—it's a little like trying to locate buried treasure in an underground cave without a flashlight—but if you have long fingers, you should curve one over the front wall of the vagina, and feel around for a little spongy pad. That's the G-spot, and when stimulated it may or may not produce a spectacular orgasm. If not, don't worry, it's perfectly alright. Some women like their clitoris played with while you have a finger or two inside them, but most will never come through vaginal stimulation alone, however hard you thrust your fingers in and out. Some even like to have a finger on or up their anus, one in the vagina, and the rest dancing around on the clitoris—but it takes a dextrous man to achieve that one without getting a hand cramp.

The basic clitoral orgasm, though, is often best achieved through accompanying nipple-stimulation. If you can tweak one with the other hand, and contrive to move you head around so you're licking the other, she may need scraping off the ceiling with a palette knife when she comes. Coming around the mountain has nothing on this one. If she merely finds three-point excitement confusing, though, stick with what you know, and keep up a gentle but steady pressure around her clitoris.

You can cup your whole hand over her pubic bone, fingers upward, and rub her slowly with the heel of it for a different kind of stimulation—but you can get more precision work in with fingertips. When she does come, take your hand away—there's nothing worse than a suddenly sensitive clitoris subjected to pressure, and she does not need a final, flourishing rub to finish with—she just needs to recover for a few minutes, till the sensitivity subsides back to normal levels. It's generally better to let her come before sex if she isn't a woman who comes through intercourse—otherwise she'll be sitting up in bed like a meerkat, waiting for her turn, and you'll be a spent, exhausted husk drifting into a coma on the other side of the bed.

touching his parts

Giving a hand job is a little like polishing a wooden banister to a gleaming shine. It's hard work, but ultimately satisfying. It's all about the grip you use—there's no immediate need for fancy techniques, though they can be highly entertaining for him—but as long as you're holding it right, he's going to come either way. Even if the house is surrounded by police cars and officers shouting through megaphones, he'll still have an orgasm before he goes out with his hands up.

the basic hand job that works—every time

To give a great hand job, you don't actually need lubrication, but it doesn't hurt—it also has the added bonus of feeling a little more like a blow job for him that way. So if you do use it, a blob the size of a nickel should do the trick, and allow your hand to slide more easily up and down his shaft. Although women like to be caressed in other areas before he heads for her parts, for men, the whole "creeping up on you gently" idea is somewhat less important. In fact, most men are likely to be attempting to nudge your hand downward shortly after "hello." So if you do want to go more slowly, just kiss him, stroke his nipples, knead his butt, and then get down there before he expires through need.

It sounds obvious, but if you're right-handed, use your right hand, otherwise your weaker arm will begin to seize up about thirty seconds before he comes. He'll be gasping and panting in ecstasy, and you'll be muttering, "I can't go on, really sorry ..." as your wrist goes limp with exertion.

Make sure you're lying comfortably so you don't have to re-arrange yourself halfway through—this is particularly important if he's touching you at the same time, of course. Now, grasp his penis with your whole hand. Too many women make the mistake of bal-ancing it as if it was a china teacup, between finger and thumb. This

---

TIP

If he's desperate for a fuck and you just want to go to sleep, it really is a kindness to offer a hand job—it's the least trouble for you, and he'll be happy and grateful. The fast-results hand job is simply a matter of expos-ing your breasts so he's got something to look at, lubricating your hand with KY, and starting fast. Forget the gradual build-up, just get a rhythm going, then go all out, swapping hands seamlessly like a drummer if your arm starts to seize up before he comes. It really shouldn't take more than three minutes—put the radio on, it's the length of a song.

When you're giving him a hand job and he starts to come, don't automatically speed up. If you go against that instinct, and continue rubbing slowly—about one stroke a second, instead of the average three a second that orgasm normally encourages—it will deepen and prolong his orgasm. He'll still come, but it will be a much slower sensation. Obviously, he'll be throwing himself around, trying to get you to speed up, so it may be worth explaining your cunning plan to him first, and seeing whether it works for him.

may eventually make him orgasm, but it will take a couple of days. You need to wrap your fingers around it with your thumb at the top, encircling the head, so just enough is poking out to enable you to rub up and down freely. Your fingers should be curved around back toward yourself, so the whole shaft is enclosed in your fist. Grip as though you mean it, but not hard enough to cut off his blood supply. A penis can take a lot more pressure than a clitoris, so don't be afraid to be firm.

Begin with a steady pace, making sure the foreskin pulls up over the head, and rolls back without impediment—if he's circumcised, you may need more lubrication. As he gets more excited (in about three seconds, usually), speed up your pace as if you're polishing that banister and the master of the house is walking down the hall toward you, about to check it for reflective sheen. Just as you get so fast you know your arm can't take the pain, he will almost certainly come—try to angle his penis so it comes all over his chest rather than your hair.

And obviously, be careful, in your excitement, not to wrench it wildly to the side. (I won't go into the potential consequences, but

TIP

Another suggestion for a memorable hand job—the "countdown" stroke—does not involve trying to make a new word out of the letters "p-e-n-i-s e-x-t-e-n-s-i-o-n." It is simply counting down hand strokes—with lubrication, give his penis nine strokes down, then nine up, followed by eight down, eight up, seven up … yes, well, you get the idea, right down to zero. After which, you can shout "blast off!" and proceed to do something even more explosive, whether that's a blow job or sex in the wheelbarrow position (with the proper protection, of course) … this stroke gets him right in the mood for it, and thoroughly builds up his excitement.

let's just say they end up on the kind of e-mail attachments bored guys send to their office-bound friends. Not pretty.)

To enhance the experience—not that it really needs it—some men like to have their balls stroked or, ideally, sucked, while you rub his penis. Make sure you can cope with multi-tasking, though, otherwise it's like rubbing your tummy and patting your head, and can result in utter confusion. If that's too much trouble, then suck or stroke his nipples as you go, or kiss his neck. As you approach the home stretch, and if your guy is the liberal sort, you can slide a finger into his anus because this will stimulate his prostate gland and result in a wildly intense orgasm for him. Afterwards he may say, "What the hell, why was your finger up my ass?" But by then, he'll be more than aware of the positive benefits of doing this.

If you want to caress his penis in a teasing fashion before you actually perform the full hand job experience, you need to focus on the frenulum—this is the tiny bit of skin that connects the head to the shaft, and responds well to very gentle stroking. Circle your fingers on the tip, then run them along the shaft, alongside the vein that runs up the front of his erect penis. Pay attention to his balls—never squeeze them, think of them as baby breasts, and treat them as you would wish your own breasts to be treated. Unless, of course, you get off on the idea of having them bitten really hard.

Don't ignore the perineum—this is the bit of skin that connects his balls and his ass, and in itself connects to the prostate gland—so light pressure on this area will, again, intensify the sensations he's feeling. That would be "light" pressure, however. Whatever you do, don't get overexcited and start beeping away at it like it's a car horn.

advanced techniques

For those who mastered the basic hand job years ago, there are certain techniques that can enhance the whole thing—as taught by Lou Paget, Californian sex educator and best-selling author, and queen of the hot move. They may take a little practice to perfect—Lou likes to allow her subjects to work on a lifelike latex penis, but you may be reduced to trying out your moves on a large cucumber if you're unsure about the real thing. Still, once mastered it's like riding a bike—you'll never forget it.

the basketweave

Link your fingers together, so both hands are clasped around his shaft—you need lubrication for this, it makes the whole thing ten times easier—then push both hands down to the bottom of his shaft, twist them, and come back up, twist at the top, go back down. As he approaches orgasm, you can get less sophisticated. But grown men may well buy you diamonds for your ability to perform this maneuver.

the heartbeat

Again, clasp your hands—but this time, as you go up and then down the shaft, "pulse" your hands in and out by squeezing lightly, moving up or down the shaft without rotating. This will mimic the sensation of you tightening around him when he is inside you. He's unlikely to come this way, but who cares when it feels so nice?

the figure eight

One-handed, perform the basic hand job, but when you reach the top and bottom, give a gentle twist each time. This activates the nerve endings of his penis that wouldn't normally get in on the action—and it's easy to do, which is a bonus.

2   positions

Having sex is easy. But having sex so you want to keep doing it with the same person is a little more difficult. While some of that may be down to how they look, and whether they smell of Givenchy Pour Homme or an overflowing ashtray, an awful lot is down to the position you choose to have sex in. There's something to be said for missionary, but sadly, that something is likely to be "effective but dull." Which means that for genuinely good sex, you need a repertoire of different positions, all of which will result in a happy sexual experience.

I could tell you all sorts of things about the Congress of the Water Buffalo, or how to make love hanging upside down from a rope, but it wouldn't be that much fun to actually put into practice. The pictures would be amazing, but the experience itself would definitely come under "once only." So the first basic question when it comes to finding a new and interesting sexual position is "is it comfortable?" and the second basic question is "is it enjoyable?" Only when the answer to both questions is "yes" should you proceed.

It's perfectly possible to have enjoyable and orgasmic sex without throwing each other around like Russian shot-putters. There are over a hundred positions that you could possibly contort yourself into—but the real question is, why would you want to? If it's not working for one of you, it's a dud. So while he may be having just the best time ever with your legs behind your ears and your head wedged between his thighs, if you feel like a human pretzel, an orgasm will be a distant dream.

TIP

A useful sexual position, though it sounds appalling, is The Clamp. You lie in the standard missionary position, then while he penetrates you, bring your legs together so the base of his penis is trapped between your thighs, and his legs are straddling yours for a change. This significantly increases the amount of friction on his penis, while your clitoris benefits from the extra pressure, too. The difficulty is, he's more likely to fall out while thrusting, and there's nothing more painful than a mis-thrust penis. Still, it's worth doing now and then, if only for the novelty value of swapping your usual leg positions around.

positions that work

Certain positions will always offer a good time. Once you have them in your arsenal, sex becomes a far more enticing prospect, because you automatically know what's going to give your clitoris the best pressure, or where you need to put your legs to activate your G-spot. Forget the *Kama Sutra*—it may have had some decent pictures if you were a love-starved ancient, but for today's couple, trying to arrange yourselves into anything similar is like trying to assemble IKEA flat-pack furniture in the dark without a screwdriver.

There are, however, a few positions that work for almost everybody, regardless of yogic ability. The most popular—assuming anybody tells the truth in sex surveys—are woman on top, and missionary. But as we're trying to make life more exciting, we'll leave missionary till later, and concentrate on The Ten Positions that Always Work. At least they do unless you've just had a fight, developed a migraine, or recently had back surgery.

the ten positions that always work

spoons

The Spoons position is the easiest and simplest of all sexual positions. All you do is lie on your side, with him behind you. He shunts up so his penis is aligned with your parts, like a spaceship docking—it helps if you both bend your legs and tuck into each other, with his arm around your waist so his hand can cup your breast. His other arm can lie along your back, or form a pillow for your head. Push your butt into his groin until your genitals are properly aligned—then in it goes. Leverage for thrusting is provided by the fact that he's holding your waist. This is a handy position for stimulating the front wall of your vagina, where the elusive G-spot may reside. It's not so good for your clitoris—unless before entering, he uses his penis tip to arouse you, while you clamp it between your thighs, ensuring that he has an equally good time.

scissors

Easier to perform than describe, the Scissors maneuver starts with you lying side by side, facing each other. Now listen carefully. You put one leg over his outer hip, and he grabs your butt. This enables him to penetrate you effectively, while you use your leg as a lever to help him thrust. He can also lick your breasts (or if he's of a mind to, he can stick his head between them and go "bbbbbbfffllbb," but you may not want him to, of course). You need to keep your bottom leg pressed against his, while your top arm goes around his waist. Look, it's really not that complicated, but of course feel free to practice with dolls first.

The bonus here is that his groin rubs your clitoral area, and you can kiss. It's also perfect placement for getting a finger up his ass, just before he comes.

doggy

Ask any man his favorite position for a full-on sex-fest fuck, as opposed to the lovey-dovey romantic kind, and if he doesn't say "doggy," he's almost certainly lying. This is possibly the sexiest position ever invented, but sadly, some women feel it's a little demeaning. It can be, if he's behind you snarling, "I don't wanna see your face bitch, I just want you to bark." But assuming he isn't, then it's simply a great experience for both of you, as far as sensation goes. Alright, yes, you may sacrifice a little intimacy, but he can always look into your eyes later on, once the excitement's died down. All you do is get

---

TIP

Men are visual little creatures, so actually seeing you while you're having sex is fairly high up on his wish-list. But even better is watching himself have sex—with you, naturally. The best sex to watch in front of a mirror is either doggy style or standing up, both of which enable you to twist your heads to look, or give you the chance to do it while facing the mirror. The standing-up position is best with a full-length mirror that's on the wall next to you. You lean forward against the wall that's at right angles (look, it's really not as complex as it sounds), while he enters you from behind holding onto your waist, giving you both a fantastic view of his penis and your ass. If you're naked, you even get to see breasts, too.

---

on all fours and stick your ass in the air. This is not dignified. But for your watching partner, it's deeply sexy. He enters you, holding on to your hips or waist, and can reach around to your breasts and clitoris. His penis will go in very deeply. It will hit your G-spot because the tight fit of entry from behind means all the vaginal nerves are touched. If you lie down with your butt still sticking up, the stimulation is even greater, and if you do it in front of a mirror, it's a great sight for both of you—it's about the only position in which you can both watch without cricking your necks.

cat

This is missionary with a much higher chance of female orgasm. If you have always orgasmed perfectly in missionary position before returning to your knitting and bible study, then ignore this bit—but if you like the intimacy and closeness of him on top, but resent the fact that he gets to come like an express train, while you're left checking his butt for pimples, this is for you. The Coital Alignment Position is simple. He lies on top of you, penis inside you, as usual—then he inches up your body till he's as high as he can get, without bending his penis agonizingly. Then, instead of thrusting, he simply grinds in small circles. A lot of good sex relies on small circles, and this is just one example. This has the effect of stimulating your clitoris thoroughly, because he's moving right on top of it continuously—with normal missionary, he's just intermittently banging it, which is going to result in nothing more earth-shattering than painful genitalia.

Your orgasm relies on him grinding slowly—as soon as he gets overexcited, it's all over. So play with his balls, kiss him—anything to distract him from the desire to get all jiggy.

face to face

Now we're getting all *Kama Sutra*—this position looks exactly like a 16th-century wood-carving and is elegantly symmetrical, compared to the wham-bam nature of most sexual couplings. All you have to do is sit facing him, on his lap. You wrap your legs over his hips and join your feet behind his butt to stay in place. He joins his feet so his legs provide a balancing platform for you. Once his penis is inside you, just rock, using his hands on the bed for balance if necessary—yours will be around him. It's the perfect position for kissing, he can reach your breasts, and your clitoris is stimulated by the pressure of his pubic bone. Admittedly, if you thrust too hard, there is a chance of tipping over—but if you keep it slow and steady you can both build up to a thrilling climax. It also allows for a lot of neck-kissing, which is one of the most erogenous zones for both of you. Just be careful not to bang teeth when it gets passionate.

standing (backward)

Standing-up sex can be a gateway to a world of disaster. If you aren't the right heights for it, you're basically a chihuahua barking up a redwood. However, there is a way around it—apart from high heels. If you're after a quickie, and lying or sitting down just isn't a possibility in the dark alleyway you've found yourselves in, then you just turn around to face the wall, stand about two feet away from it, and stick your butt out. He may have to bend down a little if your height discrepancy is big, but it's much easier for him than front-ways—if you try that, you have to get one leg up around his waist so he doesn't slip out, and stand on tip-toe, which might work for a trained ballerina but is something of a ligament-strain for the rest of us. This way, you have a wall to brace yourself against so he can thrust much harder, and better still, he can actually locate the right part without too much trouble and knee-bending. Again, it's good for your G-spot, and allows him to reach your breasts—if you have time, before the policeman points his flashlight at the pair of you.

squatting

You thought doggy was undignified—this position makes it look like a Sothebys antiques auction in comparison. But it's worth it. Basically, he lies on his back, and you squat above him. Yes, squat. Then he penetrates you, and you raise yourself up and down, using your hands on the bed—or his chest—for leverage. Don't lean forward, and you must balance on your feet, not kneel down. Yes, it will resemble constipation, but the idea is, you're at such a level of passion that neither of you will make that connection. At least, not at the time. The beauty of this position is that it instantly provides full penile access to every area of your vaginal nerves. And as you plunge up and down—because that's what you need to do—with every thrust, they'll be stimulated beyo1nd your wildest imagination. It works—you just look, on some basic level, slightly stupid. But he won't care. And from the throes of your orgasm, neither will you. It allows him room to play with your breasts and clitoris—though he shouldn't do that while you're plunging or someone could have an eye poked out.

half off the bed

Some sexual positions require some sort of prop—even in cave times, they may have done things with bison bones that we don't even want to think about. But for this one, you only need the very basic prop of a bed. You lie on your back, with your butt on the edge of the bed, and your legs on the floor. He stands up, and you wrap your legs around his waist, or at least hook your knees over his hips. He then holds your thighs, and thrusts into you, which allows for very deep penetration, and hard, passionate sex. The good part is, you hardly have to do anything, and he does all the work. He's pumping like a piston engine, you're lounging around—sounds good to me. It's a good G-spot position, too, because his penis will be rubbing against the front wall of your vagina, and again, it allows for lots of breast access. If you turn over and kneel up, his standing thrust will give you a uniquely pleasing take on the doggy position, too. The only thing required is some stamina on his part—he has to be the kind of man who doesn't go weak and jello-legged due to exertion, or else you'll be collapsing in a feeble heap after two thrusts.

legs on shoulders

This is a great position all around, but only if you're slightly flexible. If you're not, you're looking at a locked back and a lot of tears and accusations, so you may want to do some stretching exercises first to ensure suppleness. Again, you lie on your back (there's a pattern beginning to emerge here ...) and he kneels between your legs. Then you raise your legs so your ankles are on his shoulders—unless you're a giantess, they'll fit perfectly, just make sure you don't kick him in the ear when he starts thrusting. He has full access to breasts and clitoris, and you can go as fast or as slowly as you like in this position. He can hold your butt to enable thrusting, or caress you. It's best if you don't attempt to do a whole lot, given that you're doubled up at the waist like a pocket-knife, so your job is just to lie back and enjoy it. The angle again gives a great depth of penetration and because he

You should never be embarrassed by the noises your body makes during sex because men find them highly erotic—any squishy noises are part of the whole experience. You can get a similar effect from lubrication on your hands, so if you are using it, it doesn't hurt to rub them together first. Other noises—such as the charmingly named "pussy fart"—are simply a result of having air forced into your vagina by his thrusting, and therefore nothing to be embarrassed about. In fact, if it's anyone's fault, it's his.

can see all your parts, it's a visual turn on for him. You can place your feet against his chest, too, to brace against thrusting, but if you do, remember to take your high heels off first, unless you want to end the session cutting up bits of bandage and apologizing profusely.

her on top

It's old, it's familiar—but it works, without a doubt. The only negative when it comes to this position is the fact that you actually have to make some effort. This time, it's him lying back like Cleopatra on a burnished barge while you get down to the serious thrusting. But the advantage is, you get to control the pace—sometimes guys go way too fast because they get all excited, bless them. For you, there's no danger of over-thrusting, it's just a matter of which position presses best on your clitoris. Try leaning forward slightly to grind your pubic bones together, or backward if you want to expose it for rubbing. You can even rub it yourself if he isn't doing it to your satisfaction—or whip out a vibrator, and hold it between you, which is always a winner, whatever position you happen to be in. With you on top, you get great breast access, and he can fondle your ass. As you speed up, make sure you don't raise yourself too far before you plummet back, or you could miss altogether and do horrible things to his penis. Not desirable. Still, being on top allows you to rub and grind as much as you like—whereas a lot of positions mean you're in his hands as to speed and direction, this one enables you to control the pace to your precise specifications, which means you can also come when you like, roll off and fall asleep. It's only fair.

Now, with that repertoire of ten you could probably keep yourselves happy on a desert island for quite some time. But on a desert island you wouldn't have any props to enhance the experience with—so for a really good time, you'd ideally want a few ways of livening up the basic ten, with the odd twist here and there. So you may wish to investigate the following—and if you fall and break your ankle it's no use suing me, I'm only telling you, not advising you …

advanced

chair

A simple chair can make all the difference to your sexual experience—but make sure it's a non-staining fabric. The ideal kind is a solid wooden kitchen chair that isn't going to tip over the moment you get giddy. He sits on it, and you sit on his lap, facing him. He's supported with his feet on the floor, and you are supported by him holding you up. You rock, holding onto the back of the chair (don't even think about trying this on a stool, it will end in definite disaster)—he can't move much, but again, you get to control the pace, and grind your clitoris into him, which works nicely. You can try this with a rocking chair as well, but be careful you don't both go flying during a particularly passionate session.

swing chair

This is a bizarre contraption rather like the kind of thing James Bond villains have hanging in their mountain lairs, but having said that, it can offer a brand new take on the whole sex thing, and given that people have been doing it for several millennia now, that can't be bad. This swinging hammock with holes and straps hangs from the ceiling, and one partner sits in it while the other takes the opportunity to swing them around, thus gaining access to whichever orifice suits their liking. It removes troublesome gravity from the situation, so it resembles having sex in space, but without the capsule food, or oxygen problem. Once again, "dignified" isn't the word that springs to mind—but then, who cares when he has access to every single part of you, and can swing you around like some pornographic astronaut? The only drawback is you'll have to tell your mom it's a new ergonomic design when she comes to visit.

inversion

This position requires some gymnastic ability, but it's worth practicing for the head-rush you get. You know how really, really stupid and/or reckless people believe that asphyxiation leads to a stronger orgasm? Well, this is the safe version where you don't die at the end. He sits on the edge of the bed, and you sit on his lap, facing him. Then you bend backward, so your head is hanging down, and all the blood rushes to it. Make sure he's holding onto you tightly, though, or your giddy experience will revolve around the fact that he's just slammed your head into the parquet flooring. Don't attempt full sex in this position—you will get very dizzy indeed—but bending backward as an orgasm approaches should ensure an extra rush. Don't try him in the same position, however—you won't be able to hold him up and it will end up with him nursing a lump that won't be in his pants.

actual swing

Some people swear by a real swing for their kicks. If you have sex on a swing—while swinging, obviously—the G-force rush as it flies up and down can intensify your orgasms. The main thing to be aware of is who's holding on—if both of you rely on the other, you'll be swinging straight into the emergency room without looking down. Ideally, he should hold the chains, while you straddle him, and hold onto him. You can't thrust much either, and unless you have a swing on your own private land—or in the bedroom—you do run a heavy risk of being arrested by an irate park ranger.

table

Far safer, the sturdy table is an ideal sexual prop. You can use it in the same manner as the bed, but you'll get a lot more friction out of it, as the hard surface will enable you to feel every thrust much more effectively. It will also enable your butt to ache much faster, being hard wood rather than yielding mattress—but it's surely a small price to pay for kitchen-based excitement. He should stand at the end, between your legs, and you should put your feet on two kitchen chairs—or one, and wrap the other one around his waist. If you don't support your feet, your back will start to hurt, and you'll be shunting up and down rubbing sore patches on your buttocks. Most importantly, be certain it's a well-made table. You don't want everything falling apart at the climactic moment in a shower of Swedish nuts and bolts.

car

To have sex in the car, there are a variety of options (but don't do what I did once, which was leave the engine running so we could have the radio on, only to get a dead battery and end up stranded in a parking lot in the middle of nowhere at midnight …). To avoid an undignified scenario with feet sticking out of the windows of your VW Bug, you need to make sure your car is big enough. Then decide if you're going to succumb to passion in the front seats—which involves all sorts of problems with the gear shift—or climb into the back and go for it in relative comfort. The drawback of the back seat is that if you are interrupted, you have absolutely no excuse for what you were doing. Nevertheless, it's far easier to get into a relatively comfortable position, so I recommend it. He should sit upright on the back seat, and you straddle him—but only if you're not being watched. If you're next to picnicking families in a park in midsummer, you need to lie down—him along the back of the seat, and you clinging onto him like

TIP

If your relationship's gotten into a dismal rut, then sex expert Anne Hooper suggests making small changes at first that will alter the way you approach sex. So swapping the side of the bed you sleep on will automatically force a slightly different method into it, as will changing the hands you both use for hand jobs. If you wear a nightie and he wears PJs, go to bed naked, and if you always sleep naked, then wear something—ideally, something seductive. If you usually do it in the dark, switch the light on and vice versa … a change is as good as a rest, but it's also as good as a vastly improved fuck.

a baby monkey, in the Scissors position. Don't even think about reclining the front seats. It absolutely does not work.

wheelbarrow

Luckily, you do not need a wheelbarrow for this position. You do, however, need to cast your mind back to those playground wheelbarrow races, where some nine-year-old held your legs up and you staggered on your hands past the chalk markings to victory. This version, though, is even more exciting (if that were possible). For a unique sexual thrill, stand on your hands (naked, obviously) while he catches your legs, and places them on either side of his waist. Then he enters you, while holding you up. This gives him full and frank access to your entire genitalia; and you get the orgasmic head-rush from hanging upside down. You also get a locked spine, however, if you aren't damn careful, so make sure you don't attempt to hold the position for too long unless you are, in fact, a trained trapeze artiste. It does provide great access for G-spot stimulation, and if he's an ass man, he gets a great view as well.

places to do it

The obvious and easy place to explore sexual positions is in bed. But while a comfy mattress provides an ideal base, you can have a lot more fun if you use the whole house (or even street, local park, shopping center, supermarket aisle ...) as inspiration for your sexual positioning. Some places are useless, naturally, because they're too small, uncomfortable, or simply happen to be in front of your plate-glass windows that are overlooked by the neighbors (unless exhibitionism floats your boat, of course). There are, though, certain pieces of furniture or household fixtures and fittings that just lend themselves to wild sex. With the curtains drawn, obviously.

washing machine

The washing machine is a winner for sexual activity—not only can you give your dirty underwear a nice spin afterward, but you get throbbing like no vibrator ever invented, so long as you make sure to balance on it as it approaches the spin cycle. The old-fashioned type, that shudders and hums and jiggles as it cranks itself up to full power is best—that way, you get the sensation spreading from underneath your butt through your clitoris when you sit on the top and wrap your legs around his waist so he can enter you. It takes a little balance, and you must be certain it's not the kind of machine that's going to break and flood the room in your excitement—but most vital, try and time your orgasm to happen before it moves onto "final rinse" or you'll be left high and, um, dry.

TIP

At the beginning of your relationship you're up for doing it anywhere— no surface goes untried. But after a while, the bedroom is the only place that gets to see any action apart from the domestic. You have to make an effort to meet in a different venue—such as the kitchen. A simple change from the bed to the kitchen table can result in an entire range of sensations that you don't get when you're lying on a soft mattress, and lends itself to a range of new positions. But if it ain't going to happen naturally, then make a conscious decision.

---

couch

If you want a little more excitement than that dull old bed, but you don't want to get nasty carpet burns, the couch provides a great compromise. Best position is either straddling him, or doggy, lengthways on the cushions. Or you can bend over the back while he enters you from behind, or lie in missionary position and fondle his ass. Be aware, though, that it's considered terribly bad form to watch TV out of the corner of your eye while he's struggling to give you an orgasm.

kitchen appliances

Kitchen appliances are useful because they're firmly built and unlikely to collapse in the middle of your display of passion. You can perch on the edge while he stands between your legs, or lean on the counter while he enters you from behind. He can surprise you at the sink for a quickie—or more likely, you can surprise him.

shower

Having sex in water is largely overrated—it just ends up with everyone suffering from stinging eyes, and all the natural lubrication is washed away in a torrent of apricot shower gel. However, there is a way to have sex in the shower and get the whole "soaping each other sensually" excitement going, without spitting a waterfall over each other at the same time. You need to sit, though. It all goes wrong when both of you try and stand up, and is also a recipe for cracked ribs when one person slips sideways on a bath sponge. So adopt the face-to-face position, under the falling water, and rock gently—but don't use soap on each other's parts because it stings like hell.

As for having sex in the bath, two words: don't bother. No orgasm is worth the amount of heaving around you're going to have to perform to find a position that has a chance of working.

stairs

The stairs—or a flight of steps, as immortalized by Kim Basinger and Mickey Rourke in *9-1/2 Weeks*—are an interesting venue for sex. Being at different levels, they allow you to swivel your bodies around into new positions—if you're feeling wild you can hang upside down, or balance over him, as he sits down, with the higher stairs providing a handy shelf for holding on to. Of course, you may have a somewhat painful back, due to the ridges caused by lying along the stairs—but the opportunities for contorting yourselves are impressive, and it certainly adds a *frisson* to basic missionary when there's the chance you'll start sliding downward if you thrust too hard.

games

There are various sex games you can play—anything from Key Parties to Strip Chess—but the Dice Game is the best when it comes to positions.

You get two dice—for the first, write down a series of sexual positions. I suggest:

- missionary
- doggy
- spoons
- her on top
- standing up
- wheelbarrow

41

For the second, write down six venues—such as:

- kitchen table
- on the stairs
- on the washing machine
- in the car
- in bed
- on the couch

Then take turns throwing both—and the rule, of course, is that you must do exactly what it tells you. Even if that's "on the stairs, wheelbarrow." Throw again when you've either managed it or broken your ankle—whichever comes first.

3 orgasm

The orgasm is the holy grail of sex, the explosion that it all leads to, and the main cause of problems, at least as far as women are concerned. Because we're all so focused on coming, scoring the winning goal, waves crashing on the shore, wild horses galloping along the beach and every other cinematic image that was ever crassly used to suggest orgasmic union, the pressure to come—regularly and spectacularly—is enormous. The truth is, however, that most women vary when it comes to coming. At certain times of the month, generally mid-cycle, you may have wild, porn-star orgasms with the merest flicker of the clitoris—but if you're tired, stressed or pre-menstrual you can be on a chaise longue with the entire LA Lakers team and a well-thumbed sex manual and still be feeling nothing more than a faint sore patch somewhere down below.

The female orgasm is a gentle flower that needs to be unfurled slowly and kindly—of course, there will be times when you just want a violent quickie, and you may come dramatically from the sheer thrill of it all, but generally speaking, if he's giving it a couple of thrusts and then asking, "Are you close?" the whole thing will sputter out in feelings of inadequacy.

It isn't just women who suffer from orgasmic performance anxiety, either. Men, while toting their orgasmic equipment around a little more obviously, are still supposed to be able to come after a few manly strokes and all advice focuses on delaying, not speeding up, their orgasms. Nevertheless, sometimes men can suffer equally from "why isn't it happening" syndrome—tiredness, stress and drunkenness affect men, too, and his orgasm can be inhibited by any of these factors. (Of course, if you've recently said, "Hahaha, what's that pants-peanut?" upon viewing his penis, that may also explain his inability to truly let go.)

Still, the accepted wisdom is that if you rub your parts together, lick each other's parts or touch each other's parts for long enough, you will both, eventually, explode in a shower of spangles and gasping. And while that may well be the case, there are ways to ensure an orgasm is more enjoyable, less long-winded and less tension-filled for both of you.

orgasm for her

An orgasm for you, in a good 70% of cases, is down to having your clitoris stimulated. This is the bottom line, that whatever other pyrotechnics you may engage in, whatever superior brand of penis he's got, it won't make a darn bit of difference if he's ignoring your clitoris in favor of concentrating all his attempts on your vagina. While the vagina is, admittedly, great at responding, filled as it is (at least for the first 3 inches) with nerve endings, G-spots and whatnot, the clitoris is a far more sophisticated little device. While the multi-tasking vagina is there basically to let sperm in and babies out, the clitoris is the only human organ constructed solely for the pleasure of the owner. Really— there's no other reason for it than total enjoyment. If the vagina is the house, the clitoris is the wine bar next door, pumping out loud music, filled with laughing revelers having a great old time.

Many people, however intimate they've just been with their partner, avoid looking at each other when they come. It's such a deep and personal moment, it takes a lot of trust to share it. But watching your partner come is also very exciting and erotic—and can encourage your own orgasm. Tell him you'd like to look into his eyes so he doesn't shut them and turn his head away, and you must be prepared to let him do the same. You will not look silly—it'll probably be the most erotic thing he's ever seen in his life.

It doesn't just consist of the little pea-like bit you can see—it's like a baby penis, and stretches along under the skin of your labia for a few centimeters, which explains why it feels so great to have your inner labia fondled by his finger, on the way down to your vagina. The whole area is packed with nerves, too, so if he focuses on the clitoris and its immediate surroundings, he can't go far wrong. Actually he can—see "hand jobs: pressing too hard" for details—but the real mistake is dismissing the whole thing as just an unnecessary bit of skin, and going straight to the vagina without passing "Go." Of course, it plays a part—but it's not the be-all and end-all to a female orgasm.

orgasm during intercourse

Foreplay is vital for a women's orgasm—if the rest of you isn't aroused, nine times out of ten, your genitals won't be either. See "Foreplay" in Chapter 1 for details of what to do. But once you're heading down the road to sensation, it takes a big problem to set you off course. One such problem is the fact that most sexual positions fail to stimulate the clitoris steadily—so he's bashing away, wondering why you're not beside yourself with excitement, when what he should be doing is stimulating your clitoris at the same time. Now, admittedly, this takes practice. Most men are simply not dextrous enough to manipulate a clitoris sensitively while keeping up a respectable level of thrusting. So you either need to get into a position that allows him full access to rub you without any sudden jerky moves—or else you can do it yourself.

positions

Best positions are Scissors—he can reach down between your legs and it's impossible to move too fast in this position anyway—or him kneeling, you on your back with your legs spread. That way he can see exactly what he's doing, and touch your clitoris without any sudden lurching moves that are going to spoil everything. You on top can also work, if he spreads his hand on his stomach and uses his thumb to press on your clitoris as you rock.

TIP

It seems obvious—but that never stopped anybody from ignoring something. A simple but highly effective sex trick is to act like you're turned on. Presumably, you're already a little involved, or you wouldn't be there in the first place. But if you need a little extra, writhe around passionately, gasp when something feels good, and groan when it feels great. Talk to each other—saying "you're so sexy" can elevate the experience from basic sex to really great sex, simply because it makes you feel your partner's focused entirely on you. It's not about faking—just appreciating what's there more effectively.

It's possible in doggy position, but since it lends itself to urgent thrusting, it's not ideal.

diy

Of course, you could simply opt to save him the hassle altogether by touching yourself while he busies himself with the thrusting part. It may feel like he's getting off lightly (as it were) but look at it this way: you're getting touched the way you like best, and you aren't going to have to spend the whole time muttering "harder," "no, softer," "a bit to the left, please" when you're simply trying to concentrate on coming as effectively and enjoyably as possible.

There aren't many positions that don't lend themselves to a little self-starting, but it has to be said that missionary doesn't work too well. With everything else, if you can hold on one-handed, you can touch your own genitals—then he simply has to match his hip movements with your hand movements, or vice versa.

The 30% of women who do come through vaginal intercourse are usually lucky enough to have clitorises that are closer to their vaginas, so the movements inside have a ripple effect on the clit itself. Which will not happen if it's situated miles away at the top of your labia, which is more common.

the g-spot

One way of coming vaginally (if it's something you're very keen to do, of course) is to locate and utilize the elusive G-spot.

Some believe that the G-spot is merely a myth created by men (Dr. Graftenberg, to be precise) to enable them to slack when it comes to ensuring a female orgasm. If he can lie back and say, "Listen darlin I was going like a steam train and I didn't find no G-spot," then the fact that you didn't have a vaginal orgasm is in no way his fault. It's certainly worth looking for, in the way that the remains of Alexandria are worth looking for—but even if you've devoted the time, paid your teams of diving experts, and mapped what you're looking for to the last coordinate, no one's going to be at all surprised if you return empty-handed.

Still, if you're determined to mount the expedition, if you'll forgive the pun, then the basic things we know about the G-spot are these.

Some women claim they have them—but only about one in five would swear to it. It is located about 4 inches up on the front inside wall of the vagina, and feels a little spongy to the touch. To reach it—in theory—he needs to point his fingers inside your vagina toward your ass, and cup your genitals. Then he should extend one or two fingers upward, with the tips now curved over and pointing forwards to your stomach. Look, no one said this was easy, alright? Then, with a fingertip, he must search about up there until he locates the spongy bit.

Now this is where it gets more difficult. Because if his fingers aren't long enough, he can poke around up there for days and it's not going to make a bit of difference. If they are, and he magically chances upon a spot that when touched, makes you come over all hot and flushed, then, by George, he's got it. Should he find it, you'll know, trust me.

If so, he should just move the tip of his finger around very gently in—you guessed it—small circles. It will intensify your orgasm if he does this while simultaneously touching your clitoris with the other hand, in the manner of a Swiss watch-maker winding two masterpieces at once.

There are certain sexual positions that stand a fair chance of stimulating the G-spot (if it exists)—most notably, doggy position, which allows his penis to rub your front vaginal wall (and my that sounds so sexy, too …).

Your ankles on his shoulders can also work well, if he's leaning forward so his penis is pushing in and out at the right angle to stimulate the spot.

Supposedly, the G-spot orgasm will drive you insane with crashing waves of sensation—but as so few women actually know when they've had one, it may actually amount to nothing more than a pleasant sneezing sensation. Only you will know, and if it doesn't work, at least the clitoris is ready and waiting as back-up.

the a-spot

You'd be forgiven for thinking that now they're just making the damned spots up. Hey, I think I'll come up with a few … what about the P-spot halfway up the sphincter … or the Z-spot, which sends you to sleep when pressed. Still, we're nothing if not thorough, so we will accept that such a thing as the A-spot may actually exist, and go in search of it accordingly.

TIP

Lou has in her bag of tricks a Crystal Wand—a long, translucent vibrator that bends slightly at the end. The great thing about it is the little bend at the tip—which means it has a far bigger chance of actually reaching the A-, or even the G-, spot than, say, just to take a random example, his penis. So either he or you can insert it, then rotate or jiggle it gently until it makes contact with something that feels exciting. And if it doesn't, then hey, you can always use it to unclog the sink.

Lou Paget, who knows about these things, says that the A-spot is another wellspring of pleasure, at least potentially, and to find it, you must go past the G-spot until you locate a sensitive spot about an inch farther up. When stimulated, apparently, it can be responsible for the most intense vaginal orgasms. Then again, if you manage to get that far up and distinguish the A-spot from every other bit of spongy flesh up there, you probably deserve the kind of orgasm that still leaves you speechless three days later.

As far as A-spot positions go, your big chance is to shove a cushion under your ass, and place your ankles on his shoulders—so your hips are as high as they can get, and the angle of penetration is very deep indeed. And even then—well, you'll be lucky. But give it a try, you never know, right?

the u-spot

No, really, it exists … honest. And the good news is, to find this one you really don't need a fully trained Sherpa. U is simply short for urethra, and to find it just let his fingers travel a centimeter or so down from the clitoris. It's recommended that you empty your bladder before commencing the search because otherwise, the slightest pres-

TIP

For U-spot stimulation, the "frog" position is best. You should squat over him, balancing on your feet rather your knees, while he lies on his back, and rub up against the base of his penis. The U-spot is only a half-inch or so from the vagina, so this should allow it at least to make contact. You need to be in control here because the urethra is very sensitive and too much pressure can be a direct ticket to a bout of cystitis, which is no fun at all.

sure could just have you desperate to rush for the bathroom. Once you've homed in on the spot, which is right underneath the clitoris, all he has to do is stroke it lightly for those familiar old orgasmic sensations to rise up. This is a spot that comes into its own during oral sex (see below) but can be touched with his finger while he stimulates the clitoris at the same time. The position that works best here is the "frog"—back to the old undignified squat—where you crouch over him. But this time, while squatting, you lean forward slightly, so his groin is rubbing up against your U-spot—ideally his penis will be jiggling your G-spot, and frankly, the whole thing is just one big spot-stimulation.

oral for her

This is where it gets good. Oral sex is still banned in certain states—presumably because they know that when it's done right, nobody bothers going in to work, and state economics grind to a standstill. As far as good-god-I-can't-breathe-or-see orgasms go, oral sex is your best hope by a mile. The best thing about it is, you don't actually have to do anything, unless you're attempting the 69 position, which is far too complex to give you a great orgasm with ease. Most of the time, though, you're only required to lie back, legs apart, and occasionally run a hand through his hair while he licks you to giddy heights of unimaginable pleasure. At least, that's the idea. Unfortunately, however great in bed they may be, a lot of guys think that all they have to do to get you all breathless is to lick in the general area of your privates with the finesse of a Great Dane at a water bowl. And while it's hard to make being given oral sex actively unpleasant, it's not as easy as it looks to ensure it results in orgasm.

the wrong way

The wrong way for him to give you oral sex is for him to sigh, murmur, "Suppose I better," and flick your labia apart as if he's finishing off some irritating filing. Then he should definitely not proceed with a short series of giant licks, administered fairly harshly, after which he will struggle upward wiping his chin and say, "Are you nearly there?"

Men have to understand that a woman's genitals are a delicate thing, and they no more respond to violent rubbing and licking than would a kitten. Also, if you aren't feeling right mentally it's almost guaranteed you won't come through oral sex. It's so intimate and if you're feeling remotely worried about the smell, taste, look, feel or, er, sound of your most womanly parts you'll never relax enough to breathe properly, let alone come. Just remind yourself that most men are hard-wired to find the whole package desperately attractive, and if he doesn't, either you haven't washed for a good couple of weeks, or he's wondering if that e-mail attachment he opened was actually a virus, now consuming everything on his hard drive....

the right way

The right way is for him to kiss his way down your body, finally approaching your genitals as though they are the best chocolate saved from the box. Small noises of lust and appreciation work very well. He should kiss them all over, then very gently use his finger and thumb to slightly part your labia, which has the effect of exposing your clitoris more effectively, and allowing more of it to be stimulated.

Then, if he's simply opting for the basic stimulation method (see below for "Advanced Methods"), he should flicker his tongue across your clitoris and down to your vagina a couple of times, before returning to your clit and making tiny circles around it with his tongue, in a steady, gentle rhythm. He shouldn't take his tongue away at any point, and he certainly shouldn't stop to pick pubic hairs out of his teeth, which just has the effect of making him look like a 17th-century king picking wren bones from his molars.

He must just keep going, and be led by your gasps—if you push at the back of his head, he should assume you want the pressure harder, and if you pull him by the ears, he can surmise that you want it softer. He can also slide a finger into your vagina as he goes, but some women find this distracting, so be sure to tell him if his finger-work is taking your concentration off what his tongue's doing.

If he's really coordinated, he can reach up and play with your nipples—for many women this drives them completely over the edge, but only if you can shake the mental image of him being stretched on a rack as he juggles with all your parts at once. My advice: Shut your eyes, and forget what it looks like. When you come, he should be guided by you—if your clitoris has suddenly become deeply sensitive, he should move away, but not so suddenly that he's implying

---

TIP

The nipple orgasm may or may not be a myth. But just in case it isn't, the way to get one is, apparently, for him to suck gently on your tongue and lips, then exert the same pressure on your nipples, for the same amount of time. He may need to do this several times, but whether or not you actually have an orgasm, it's certainly going to feel pretty good. As a compromise, unless you have stunningly sensitive nipples that orgasm at the flick of a switch, he can also touch your clit.

"thank god that's over"—a few more little kisses in the general area should serve as reassurance.

advanced methods

the kivin method

Lou Paget has a method of oral sex that almost guarantees orgasm every time. "George Clooney and Brad Pitt come and stand naked at the end of the bed ..." (nah, just kidding). It's called the Kivin method—not the Kevin method, though you can call it that if you wish. And it's fairly simple for him to do.

There are three points he needs to focus on—the ones on either side of the clitoral hood (the little bit of skin that conceals the clitoris when it's not in use) and one on the perineum (the bit that joins your butt with your vagina). He needs to place one finger on the perineum, and move his tongue across the two points, while two fingers are held on either side to expose your clitoris.

TIP

For a higher chance of multiple orgasms, you need to practice on building up your PC muscle—the one that you stop pee mid-flow with, or unscrew bottle caps with if you happen to be an exotic dancer in a Thai bar. If you spend five minutes a day for three weeks tightening and releasing your PC muscles, this amount of practice will result in a spectacularly tightened muscle, which will result in more orgasmic sensations when he's inside you. It will also ensure you never wet yourself when you sneeze, though that's probably not a big worry for you yet.

The other difference between this and more conventional methods is that for the Kivin method, he isn't lying between your legs—instead, he's lying at right angles to your body, with his head pillowed on your thigh. This makes it less likely that he'll press too hard, and also means you can touch him more easily. In fact, it's a winner all around—and according to Lou, if he gets it right, you can have several orgasms in a row, or what's commonly known as a "multiple orgasm."

multiple orgasm

A multiple orgasm simply means having more than one orgasm in a single sex session, via whatever method happens to be available. It does not necessarily mean the biggest orgasm of your whole, entire life (see "Full Body Orgasm," Chapter 8, for details on that one).

To heighten your chances of getting more orgasmic, you'll need to tighten up your PC muscle, which is the muscle you can feel when you squeeze as if you're stopping pee from coming. To do this—also known as Kegel exercises—just locate and squeeze, in bouts of 5 minutes. Yes, alright, it's a little tedious, but no one can see you're doing it, and it tightens your vagina beautifully.

It means that you can grip his penis harder—which, in turn, means you get more friction. But more importantly, it means that when you start to come, you can use those muscles to squeeze and release several times, which will, theoretically at least, allow your orgasm to peak and dip several times before it finishes.

If you can keep going for one after another, he should let you recover for a few minutes—at least one minute, at any rate—till the extreme sensitivity subsides a little from your clitoris—then he can use his tongue to stroke gently alongside it. Extreme gentleness is the best way to get more than one orgasm—fingers are a little rough after the first; the mouth is a much better bet.

his orgasm

His orgasm is basically a whole lot simpler to deal with. The fundamental equation is, rubbing long enough = orgasm. But there are ways of doing it that will, inevitably, result in better, quicker or slower—depending on which you prefer—orgasms for him.

during sex

Orgasming during sex is, for him, the main goal—and it is, shall we say, a whole lot easier for him to come this way than it is for you. He needs simple friction against his penis, and since the vagina provides perfect friction all the way around, not to mention the warmth and wetness he's come to associate with an orgasm, it's usually inevitable that he will come. If you'd like to slow down his headlong rush to ejaculate, there are certain positions that improve his chances of hang-

---

TIP

To prolong his orgasm, and even extend it to multiple status, he also needs to work on his PC muscles. In his case, this gratifyingly involves watching him drape a washcloth over his penis and attempt to lever it up and down for five minutes a day. Hilarious entertainment though this is—and you may want to construct some rope and pulley systems where he can pull toy cars up and down—if he gets really good, it also ensures that he will last longer when he's inside you.

ing on just that bit longer. Long enough for you to start enjoying yourself, at any rate.

Deep penetration positions where he gets to thrust hard and fast are obviously no good for delaying his orgasm. The best types are those that require him to go at your pace, and can accommodate occasional stops and starts.

You on top is ideal. You can just sit there squeezing your PC muscles for a while, ensuring he still has a good time, but unless they're like a python's stomach muscles it's unlikely he'll come through this method alone. Then when you do allow him to move, you can raise yourself up slightly to stop him from penetrating you with the whole shaft, because stimulation of just the tip is also unlikely to make him explode immediately. When it's time, you can move up and down suddenly, which is almost guaranteed to have a thoroughly orgasmic effect.

Another useful position is the face-to-face; again, you're in control of the depth of penetration. If you want him to come sooner, just choose a position that allows for deep penetration and a pace that is controlled by him—missionary or doggy, for example.

intensifying it
anal parts

To intensify his orgasm, there are various tricks you can master. And a familiarity with his prostate gland is just one of them. This little bean-shaped organ is situated toward the top of his anal passage. If you aren't too squeamish about stuffing a well-lubricated finger up there, you can caress it as he thrusts, or even as you give him a blow job. Be gentle; he can be sensitive up there—but pressing lightly on it as he's about to come can noticeably increase the strength of his orgasm.

The perineum is a useful place to press, too, being rich in nerve endings, and close to said prostate—but do not press too hard or it may well all go horribly wrong, and end in tears of agony rather than gasps of excitement. Just press it as you would an elevator button— enough for it to light up, not enough for it to malfunction altogether.

Some men love the sensation of having their anus pressed while you're touching their penis or having sex—but best check first, in case he's got some deep-seated paranoia about it, and the merest brush of finger on anus results in a flaccid penis and an embarrassed man.

balls

Balls are a tragically neglected area, but they are highly sensitive little organs and should be treated with respect and affection. If you stroke his balls while you stimulate his shaft, it can make his orgasm the great-est, most contented spontaneous explosion of feeling since his favorite team won the Super Bowl. They have a little ridge running up the middle, which responds very well when stroked or licked. If you can fit one or both into your mouth (though obviously not while you're having sex), this feels fantastic for him, and will almost certainly result in spectacular orgasm if you're stimulating his penis at the same time. You can even hum on them—you may feel utterly stupid, but it will have the same effect as a small vibrator, which feels great for him.

The only thing you have to remember with his balls, though, is Tread Carefully. It doesn't matter what amazing things you're doing to the rest of him if you're being too rough with them—he will regis-ter only pain. So never bite, chew, flick, tap or squeeze them. Other than that, you're free to fondle, caress, lick, suck, stroke and blow on them with abandon, though don't be surprised when they suddenly shrink to half the size and rise upward—it simply means he's about to come.

the basic blow job

It really isn't difficult to give a blow job—at worst, it can be mildly uncomfortable—for you, not him. It's only uncomfortable for him if you clamp your teeth together while you're doing it.

All you have to do is put his penis in your mouth, and lick and suck. But if you're hoping he'll enjoy a great orgasm at the end of it, you may require a little more in the way of technique.

The best position for giving a blow job is either crouched between his legs, him sitting—a little porno-like, I know, but we're talking about what's most comfortable for you here—or lying, as he does in the Kivin method, at right angles to his body, with your head pillowed on his thigh, as he lies on his back. Never attempt to give him a blow job while lying between his legs, you'll get the most appalling crick in your neck halfway through, if not before.

TIP

If you have long hair, it's very sensual for him if you wrap strands of it around his penis and stroke it up and down over the head—you can even give him a hand job with your own hair wrapped around him for friction. The smell and texture of your hair can be a real turn-on for him—some men even have a hair fetish—so don't ignore it as a sexual tool. If you haven't got long hair, you can achieve a similar effect with a silk scarf. And it's not as difficult to wash when he comes all over it, either.

TIP

For a very dirty and porn-friendly version of sex (ideal for, say, when you've got your period) you can give him a tit job. There may be a man out there who doesn't like this, but he's probably listening to a Judy Garland album right now. So he puts his penis between your breasts, you squeeze them together with your upper arms—or if you have small breasts, your hands—and he thrusts away. You can use body oil or KY to make it smoother—and, of course, you may be able to bend your neck forward so you can lick the tip as he thrusts upward. There's every chance he'll want to come on your face—or you can be a really kind porn-star and take him in your mouth, the choice is all yours.

Begin by circling your tongue on the tip of his penis while placing your hand around the base. This is a highly useful move, as you can use this to elongate the length of your mouth—you're probably never going to get six inches in without gagging, so if three inches are being attended to by hand, it's much more manageable for your mouth, and he knows no different. Deep throating is a myth—and since the average man's penis measures 5-3/4 inches and the average woman's mouth is 3 inches, it's just as well. Now, slide your mouth over the shaft and close your lips over it, tucking your teeth firmly away. Move up and down, angling your head so you're hitting the inside of your cheek rather than your throat with the tip. Suck lightly, but not so hard it makes your cheeks ache. Occasionally flicker your tongue along the sensitive ridge that runs along the front of his penis, and pay a little attention to the frenulum with the very tip of your tongue. As he gets more desperately eager, he will thrust and leap like a spawning salmon in a bid to get farther into your mouth. Your hand will stop this from happening, so make sure you're moving it in rhythm with your mouth, and failing that, a gentle flex of the jaw can help.

The faster you go the better as he approaches an orgasm, but don't adopt such a breakneck pace you're going to collapse exhausted thirty seconds before the finishing line. Keep up a regular, steady beat, and move your hand faster rather than your neck, while increasing your sucking pressure. And he will, almost certainly, come.

You can elaborate on this blow job, but it doesn't need much embellishment, so if you feel like moving up and down flicking your tongue up and down the main vein, or twisting your head slightly as you reach the tip, to give him extra sensations, go right ahead—but if you don't, he still won't complain.

spit or swallow?

The eternal question—it's entirely up to you. But if you are going to swallow—which is nicer for him, even if it's not for you—let it hit the back of your throat, collect it all there while he finishes, then swallow it down like a teaspoon of jam. Otherwise, you'll be wondering whether you really should hate the taste quite that much, and imagining all the little baby sperms swimming excitedly down your gullet looking in vain for something to fertilize.

If you do it this way, trust me, you won't feel a thing. If you'd rather spit, you're in good company—about 60% of women are with you on that one.

multiple for men

Men can feasibly have multiple orgasms—but they generally can't ejaculate more than once so their ability to have multiples is reliant on their control of our old friend, the PC muscle. In men, this is the muscle that's working when their penis twitches involuntarily (just say "Britney" to him if you need a demonstration of this in action). If he squeezes it just as he's about to come, once it's strong enough it can actually prevent him from ejaculating—he'll experience all the rush of an orgasm without the end result—and if he has sex again shortly afterwards, he can experience prolonged orgasmic feelings. In theory, he can keep going, squeezing and starting again. So book a month or two off work if you're planning on teaching him the method.

4   spicing it up

In the first six months of a relationship, as well as laboring under the belief that you both agree on your musical tastes and could never have an argument, you're almost certainly having sex as though hell-bent on repopulating the planet in the nuclear aftermath. This is for various reasons—like you haven't yet noticed his habit of turning his boxers inside out to wear them for two days, and he hasn't chanced upon your Phil Collins collection—but more importantly you're both flooded with PEA, the Love Hormone, which tells you that you must make love 24/7 because you two are the only people on the planet who have ever understood the point of sex. This subsides after a while, because if it didn't, you'd never get any work done due to your compulsion to lick each other's crevices while other people are hunched over their desks earning money.

The trouble is, once it's worn off, you still need to like the idea of having sex. Many couples attempt all kinds of drastic things to make sure the spark doesn't flicker and die, from affairs to plastic surgery to counselling—but the good news is, there are several much easier ways of spicing up your jaded sex life without having to pay thousands of dollars in court costs and therapists' fees.

The problems usually begin when real life has intruded good and well—say, by way of children, or work, or general exhaustion—and it's perfectly common to find your partner somewhat less devastating than you did at first, once you're used to their snoring, comforter-

TIP

Men love to be surprised—so if the mood takes you, grab him when he's got nothing more sexual on his mind than cooking pasta (though in certain "specialist" shops I believe you can buy penis-shaped pasta …), undo his pants, and give him a blow job. However, do not do this a) if you're beside an uncovered window, b) if he's holding a pan of boiling water, it'll land on your head for sure, or c) if he's in a meeting at work. Other than that, go for it.

stealing ways. But as long as you still fundamentally like each other, and aren't filled with loathing over the way the other eats soup or rustles the newspaper, then it's worth pursuing a more exciting sex life, rather than giving up and running away with somebody else, with whom you'll be flooded with PEA for six months, only to realize that they steal the comforter, too.

spontaneity

Being spontaneous takes planning, right? It's all very well for sex manuals to tell you to surprise him by opening the door naked—but first you have to take a shower, shave your legs, make sure it really is him at the door, check that no neighbors are passing by, and assume that he isn't too tired to appreciate your little display. Planning is a good idea in most cases—besides, thinking about it in advance can succeed in turning you on in advance, too.

Obviously, you don't have to pre-arrange the whole thing like a military campaign, but it helps to have an idea of the mood, or what you're aiming for—it's no good presenting him with a sudden two-hour massage session if what he really wants is to watch football. If you want to be truly spontaneous, however, most men won't complain if you offer them a blow job at any time of the day or night.

On the whole, though, it pays to plan your sudden sexual moments to the point that you know you're both going to appreciate them.

Of course, this doesn't stop you from sidling up behind him and kissing his neck—we're talking about spontaneity that demands an immediate response. If he "spontaneously" books you into a hotel, that's great—but not if you'd arranged to go to a party with your best friend the same night. So small, unexpected gestures are perfect, but enormous, complicated unexpected ones are not quite so good.

planning sex

Planned sex sounds about as sexy as an gynecologist's office. Passion isn't the first word that springs to mind, it's true, when you think of pre-arranging your sexual moments—but if you leave it to chance, chance can stretch on for a good couple of months, unfortunately. By

---

TIP

Send him a series of sexy text messages throughout the day to keep him all worked up. Obviously, it helps if he knows they're from you—otherwise he might not mention them and then you'll think he's having an affair … god, it's way too confusing. But assuming he does know, just send him a few straight-to-the-point little thoughts like "want 2 fck?" or "u make me horny" or, for the shyer young lady, a simple, "can't w8 2 c u." If he comes home and says, "What were all those weird messages about?" assume he doesn't understand text language and show him what you meant instead.

agreeing that you'll devote an evening to each other, you set up a certain expectation—but not so much so that you feel like an alarm clock is hanging over your heads ready to kick into action the moment the bottle of wine's opened. You don't have to grimly agree to sex—you're just giving yourselves the opportunity to have sex should you want to. Normally you stagger to bed so tired you're lucky if you can pick up a book, let alone each other's genitals. This way, you're focused on what else you might do in bed. You can make it like a date; text him to arrange to meet him in the bedroom, and chill some wine (unless it's red, in which case it'll taste disgusting). Then you can kick off proceedings by giving him a massage and, with luck, he'll offer one in return.

After that, it doesn't take a scientist to figure out what goes where.

changing the routine

One of the most obvious problems behind sexual boredom is the fact that sex quickly becomes part of the same old routine. For a start, most couples nearly always have sex in the bedroom—which, with its peeling posters and overflowing laundry basket, is rarely the most desirable place to do it. And if you're in the same old familiar place every night, it's hardly surprising if you're having the same old familiar sex as well. It's ridiculously easy to slip into a series of well-worn moves—quick kiss, breast fondle, a play with each other's parts and straight onto intercourse, strictly in the missionary position, followed by sleep. It's a rare couple that are still bending themselves into paperclip shapes in a bid for sexual union after the first few months—after all, why bother, when simply thinking "I'll lie back and let him do the work" is so successful? Well, it's successful in that you'll orgasm because he knows exactly what to do, but it's not so good in the sense that you'll be so bored half the time you won't want to bother in the first place.

The slightest changes can have a major effect on your sexual routine because we appear to be programmed to respond to change by instigating more change. That's why middle-aged men don't just run away with their secretaries, they run away with their secretaries, and get a haircut that's too young for them, and buy a sports car they can't afford, all at the same time.

So the idea is that if you change the environment you're having sex in, your sexual routine will get a handy shake-up, too. This is certainly the case if you've decided to alter the venue to a quickie on the interstate. But as spicing it up goes, that may be pushing things a little too far. Ideally, you'll get rid of the kids/dog/friends for a night, and head straight for the nearest four-star hotel. There's absolutely no point in this whatsoever if your objective is to save money—because there's nothing less sexy than a miserable 2-star B&B, with fire regulations on the door and tattered sheets on the bed. You may as well stay at home and be uncomfortable for free.

But if you pool your resources and can afford something half-decent with a nice shiny marble bathroom and a big bed, then you're already halfway there.

Just one night should be enough to revitalize things—but make sure you order room service, or midnight will strike and you'll still be waiting in the restaurant for your coffee. Oh, and get something delicate, there's no point stuffing yourselves on a gargantuan feast, and then falling asleep.

If you really can't afford a hotel, then do something different in the house—move the furniture around, buy some new bed linen, paint the walls a vibrant shade of pink—anything that improves the sex quotient of your bedroom. Hell, you could even consider not letting the dog sleep on the end of your bed—it's all very cozy, but it's also slightly unsettling when Sadie the spaniel is gazing at you in innocent horror as you attempt to have a good time.

clothing

Along with changing the environment, you may wish to think about changing what you wear to the boudoir. That worn-out old Mickey Mouse T-shirt you've been sleeping in for years may be cozy, but it ain't screaming "Marilyn Monroe," is it? Now, I don't care how much of a card-carrying feminist you are, I'm one, too, but that doesn't mean you have to dress like something out of *Maxim*. Men are highly visual creatures, configured to respond instantly to an attractive sight—and you in decent lingerie comes somewhere near a double overtime football win on his mental list of attractive sights. You may prefer the sensible white bra and panties combo, but rest assured, nine men out of

---

TIP

Showering can be as dull and functional as teeth-cleaning. But it doesn't have to be. Next time he's singing in the shower, jump in there—naked, dummy—and give him a full and thorough washing. Remember, though, if you do intend to move on to full sex, don't attempt it standing up—it'll all end in disaster. Just use your skills with the soap to make sure he's clean in every nook and cranny. Ideally, you'll use unscented shower gel—otherwise it can all get horribly stingy in his (and your) most intimate areas.

Don't leave sex till the evenings—you're both tired. Studies show that afternoons are the best time to have sex because that's when they're at a peak. So what better way to liven up the day than to take an extended lunch hour and lure him home from work? You can always invent an urgent dental appointment. For both of you. A lunchtime quickie makes life so much more exciting than a weary roll just before sleep overtakes you— and you'll both go back to work feeling great. If you make it back, that is.

ten prefer skimpy, black, lacy stuff, given the choice. And the tenth is just temporarily lost in some virgin-deflowering fantasy.

You don't have to spend fortunes on nice underwear—it's not going to be on that long. But you need a bra (avoid heavily padded cups, it's only disappointing for everyone when it comes off), a G-string (unless you have a mammoth-sized butt, in which case French panties are a good bet), a garter belt (yes, I know, fiddly, time-consuming, pointless, but will drive him wild) and stockings. All men like stockings, particularly black ones. Don't think you'll meet him halfway and wear knee-highs, incidentally—knee-highs are the death of sex. You can also add high heels, and don't complain you'll look like a hooker—that's the point. It isn't giving in to the forces of sexist evil, it's just giving him a good time, and it's not as if he's really paying you. Chance'd be a fine thing. Dressing up shows you care about his enjoyment, and more importantly, that you still view yourself as a sexual being, which is a turn-on for you and him. Trudging to bed in frayed underwear that say "Monday" on the front (particularly when it's Thursday) and one of his T-shirts does not suggest that you see yourself as anything other than a person who happens to sleep in the same bed as him.

Of course, he must return the favor by ensuring that he doesn't wear comedy boxer shorts from six Christmases ago and that his underwear is clean, attractive and in no way bears a resemblance to something a male lap-dancer might wear. Boxers or trunks are harmless, lycra speedos are not.

It goes without saying—almost—that hygiene should be of impeccable standards for both of you. But somehow I suspect he may need reminding slightly more often than you do.

stripping

Right, now forget you ever were a feminist for a moment, and consider making your partner dizzy with gratitude—by learning how to strip. Wrenching off your clothes at the end of the day and shouting,

---

TIP

Men are visual creatures, we all know that, so what better visual thrill than you in underwear, or even naked? And to make it more exciting than the "you in underwear" he gets to see every single night when you're chucking clothes on the bed, make it a surprise. Tell him you're "just stepping upstairs to get something" while he's comatose in front of the TV ... then reappear five minutes later in your best and sexiest lingerie and high heels. Naturally, he will understand your intentions immediately. Unless football's on, in which case he might murmur, "Are you hot or something?" without taking his eyes off the tube.

A simple but effective tip—always dim the lights, or switch lamps on, when you're in the mood. There's nothing more passion-killing that a great big 100-watt bulb beaming down on you, highlighting every lump and bump and making the pair of you look like plucked turkeys ready for Christmas dinner. It might make you hungry, but it certainly won't make you horny. A couple of lamps in the corners should cast the sort of flattering glow that makes you look like a honey-skinned beauty, and create enough shadow to make the room look vaguely sensual rather than like an operating theater.

"OK, I'm off for a shower," as he briefly glances up from the paper is not stripping.

Seductively removing each and every garment while gyrating to a suitably sultry tune and taking his breath away in the process, however, is.

Helen Jackson, an ex-stripper, runs classes, and has boiled the Perfect Strip down to a series of winning moves. With her expertise behind you, you won't feel stupid, clumsy or embarrassed; you will simply feel like a goddess luring him to your temple. Or at least, you'll feel quite sexy, and that can only be a good thing, right?

Wear a long dress that's easy to undo—no stripper ever looked good getting out of a polo neck and jeans. Under it, you need the full lingerie experience, plus elbow-length gloves and high heels.

Choose your music—something with a good beat, but not too fast. Begin by standing with your feet together, sticking your butt out—think Bunny Girl.

When you're performing your striptease—or simply seducing him—it's vital that you show yourself off to the best advantage. So wear a high-cut G-string or panties (high cut up the legs, that is, not the butt) to elongate your legs and make you feel tall and slim. Don't believe that stuff about hip-huggers "giving you shape"; most men would infinitely rather look at you wearing panties that are held together by dental floss than admire the "shape" created by large lycra undies. Bridget Jones did not know what she was doing when it came to seduction—you, however, do, and all you have to remember is, the skimpier the better.

Now place your hands in the small of your back, so you're pushing out your breasts and butt simultaneously.

Dance for him for a little while (note: playing air guitar does not count and ruins the atmosphere). Keep eye contact—and don't laugh. In fact, to avoid untimely giggling you may want to have a glass or two of champagne before you begin to get in the mood.

Make him believe you're about to remove a garment—and then take your hand away again .... Start with your gloves. Pull each finger out, one at a time, taking four steps between each pull—then whisk the whole glove off and throw it to him to catch. He isn't allowed to touch you—so keep coming close then backing off. Unzip your dress and let it fall off your shoulders, pull it back up, turn around away from him and then let it drop to the floor.

Kick it aside, drop your bra straps, pull them back up … you get the picture. Every time you take something off, turn away, then turn back with your hands covering your body.

Flash your breasts at him and then cover them again … and wear high-cut underwear, because they make your legs look extra long. You may wish to leave your shoes and stockings on—if not, make sure you wear thigh-highs, and slowly roll them down.

Finally, when you're naked, keep your arms by your sides, pushing your cleavage together, jut one hip out … and after that, it's open season.

Of course, he could return the favor by stripping for you. And indeed, if you like that sort of thing, go ahead. But to many minds, the sight of a grown man gyrating to sappy music while sliding his zipper up and down, is just plain old stupid, unless he's being paid to do it for a bachelorette party. So perhaps leave the stripping to those who know what they're doing, i.e., you.

danger

There is a pretty foolproof way of spicing up your sex life—risking your life. Scientific studies have proven that the closer you come to danger, the more sexually aroused you are directly afterwards. So you

---

TIP

Call him at work and suggest he joins you for a "quick lunch." Say you've got something you want to ask him—though you may want to add that it's not "can we have a baby," "can we move in together" or "let's get married"—delete as appropriate. When you meet—whether that's at home or in a restaurant—say, "About what I wanted to ask you … want to fuck?" and lead him to the nearest bed/bathroom stall/backseat of car. This is when quickies really come into their own.

TIP

Putting your leg up on a chair—or his lap—is a highly seductive move, as utilized by pole-dancers the world over, because it makes your legs look longer by tightening your thigh muscle, shrinking your butt, and it makes you bend forward to show off cleavage. If you wear a long skirt with a split in it, which you can contrive to have fall open at the crucial moment, so much the better. And if you're not wearing anything, you get the picture. Just don't expect him to be able to breathe for a good hour afterward. If you're wearing high heels, though, a piece of advice—watch where you place your stiletto.

perform a bungee jump, and seconds afterwards, you're ready to fuck like there's no tomorrow—adrenaline is belting around your blood-stream, you're flooded with the joy of living, and the first thing you want to do is share your seed, or eggs, with the nearest person. So if you and your partner share a scary experience that gets your hearts pumping and your hormones racing then you're much more likely to cling passionately together afterwards than you are if you've shared nothing but a TV dinner and a beer.

Obviously, major lifetime scary experiences aren't that useful for your sex life—canoeing down the rapids of the Colorado River might be fantastic, but it's not the kind of thing you can do when you fancy a midweek fuck. A good horror film (try *The Others* on DVD, I nearly cried with fright) or an exciting sports event—the provision being that you both have to genuinely find it exciting—may well have a positive effect on your libidos, and revitalize your emotional responses. And if not, hey, you'll have something to talk about at the office tomorrow, even if it's not your sex life.

If horror movies don't float your boat, then consider having risky sex. Not the kind you have with a Brazilian transvestite named Venus and a shared syringe full of heroin. The kind where you could get caught. That's "could," though, not "probably will," you'll note. So doing it in the back of a rented limo with a sliding screen is, for instance, better than doing it in the back of a taxicab with a greasily fascinated driver. And doing it in a deserted woodland is better than doing it in the grounds of a crowded national park on a Sunday afternoon. The mere suggestion of "someone could, potentially, come past and spot us ..." is enough to add a *frisson* of extra excitement to your jaded sex lives. But don't let that *frisson* develop into a policeman and his three giggling sidekicks, will you?

Good places include deserted parking lots (without security cameras), beaches, other peoples' bathrooms at parties, and nightclub restrooms at that stage of the evening when several people crowding into one stall is far from uncommon.

TIP

If talking dirty is a little embarrassing—and you live on your own together—get some sex fridge magnets. They enable you to spell out the filthiest comments—and even poems—imaginable, without ever actually having to voice your dirty sentiments. You can construct entire porn short stories on the fridge ... but don't do what a friend of a friend did. Feeling frisky, he composed several thoroughly X-rated odes to his girlfriend's intimate loveliness and left it there for her to find next day. Forgetting, of course, that the cleaner was due at 9:00 a.m. Who took it personally and promptly resigned ... oh well, can't win 'em all.

being sexy

underwear: lack of ...

Being sexy is about more than simply leering, "Alright sailor, what about it?," although there are certain situations where that can be a good start. But in a long-term relationship it requires a little more effort. Going out without panties on is a good start, but remember to mention to him that you—oops!—forgot your underwear. Otherwise you'll just spend the night wriggling uncomfortably and he'll wonder why you appear so distracted. It helps if you wear a skirt that's short enough to be suggestive but long enough to stop you from getting arrested for indecent exposure. He could go out without underwear, too, but should he get an erection at an unfortunate moment, he's doomed, and will have to spend the remainder of his evening out with coats piled in his lap.

mirrors

If that seems a little too exposed, investigate the erotic potential of mirrors. Not on the ceiling, unless you suffer Bond-esque delusions—but a mirror positioned so you can see yourselves cavorting on the bed doubles your erotic fun. Anyone with the slightest hint of narcissism can get off on looking at themselves having abandoned sex, and if you don't think you're so hot, you can get a whole new view of your partner—when else do you get to see their ass thrusting into you? Oh, of course, the gang-bang video you made last New Year ... but apart from that?

food

Eating food off each other is a perfect way to spice up your sex life. There are, of course, certain foods that lend themselves to sexual shenanigans. Hot food doesn't generally come into this category—no one ever ate stew off each other convincingly. You might get away with melted chocolate, though.

The ideal eating-off-people food is fruit, being as it is clean, sweet and easy to eat in one bite. Alright, yes, it's a bit of a cliché, but if it didn't work, it wouldn't have become a cliché, think of that. Fruits you desperately need to stock up on for your night of—and I'm not going to sink so low as to say "fruity passion"—love include strawberries, grapes, melon (in handy bite-sized chunks), raspberries and, of course, bananas. The banana is for obvious reasons (no, not to compare his penis against ...), but if you are going to insert it into yourself, try not to let it break off before he eats it out of you.

TIP

Go supermarket shopping and fill a basket—or if you're feeling really frisky, a whole cart—with foods you can eat off each other, or out of each other (banana-filled nostril, anybody?). Suggestions include fruits such as strawberries, bananas and grapes, chocolate, honey, even licorice whips to tie in bows around his penis if you so desire. You can also add ice cream, champagne, chocolate liqueur, puddings in your favorite flavor ... just don't eat so much that you're too full to move. That's kind of not the point.

> **TIP**
>
> Food and sex are ideal for those who aren't too uptight about a mess. If you are, you may as well forget it because you'll never enjoy it. You're way too worried about sticky substances left on sheets for it to be worthwhile. Otherwise, you can just make sure you've got old sheets on the bed and stick them in the washer afterward. Do not, however, think you'll leave on the new Calvin Klein comforter and "just be careful"—it'll be carnage, and the chocolate stains will never come out, so be warned.

Pineapple rings are also nice to balance on his penis, though if they actually fit over it, you're in trouble, size-wise. And be careful you don't get so absorbed in eating it you ignore the whole point of the exercise.

You can also involve liquids in your world of edible pleasure—champagne can be poured over each other and licked off, and it has the added bonus of smelling and tasting fantastic as well as getting you drunk and enabling your inhibitions to disappear entirely. You may think you shouldn't be inhibited with a long-term partner, but the more of a domestic life you lead, the harder it can be to let go of all your mental lists about taking the garbage out and paying the newspaper boy, and actually immerse yourself in simply being sexual. So yes, alcohol can help. But you obviously didn't hear that from me.

If you are using champagne, be aware that the bubbles can sting like hell on your most personal parts—it's OK for him, as long as you don't pour it in the top, owwwwwww! The best way is to fill your mouth with liquid, close your lips over the top of his penis, and swoosh it around, before swallowing and commencing a blow job. He'll be your slave—at least for five minutes.

He can do the same for you, licking it—quickly—out of your labia before it starts to sting. Or if that's too hardcore, off your breasts.

Tea and coffee are ideal blow job material—forget all that nonsense about ice cubes, just take a mouthful of hot (not boiling) liquid and repeat the champagne-swoosh maneuver.

Anything you ever read about or saw in a Madonna film involving hot wax—forget that as well. It just hurts.

Honey is a great food for licking off each other—it's tasty, sterile and, apart from the ruined fixtures and fittings, it's convenient, particularly when you buy it in squeeze bottles. But don't pour it on one another's hairy parts, it's a little too unpleasant to get out of the roots. As for peanut butter, it might be more trouble than it's worth. Yogurt is like being in bed with some wholefood-eating hippie (plus it smells funny), ice cream is too damn cold (though you can alternate a mouthful of ice cream and a mouthful of hot tea on the nipples/genitalia for a reasonably exciting effect), and cream has the same smell problem as yogurt. So don't bother stocking them in your erotic larder.

TIP

According to a scientific study, women are turned on by the smells of cucumber and licorice, and for men, pumpkin pie is a sensory excitement beyond measure. Don't even begin to ask me why, but the smells honestly send more blood to the genitals, thus sensitizing them further. So try burning a cucumber-scented candle, or using Demeter cucumber perfume on your wrists for a sensual charge. And it's surely possible to find something pumpkin-pie scented without having to cook the damn thing yourself.

Vegetables must, of course, get a mention. But only in the sense that if you want to do each other with carrots, that's entirely your business. Vegetables are not fundamentally sexual objects, but if you can find ways to press an eggplant—or, for that matter, a cucumber—into service, then you go right ahead and do that. But make sure it's damn clean first—or possibly even peeled. But not diced, of course.

quickies

If you have hours at a time to devote to vegetable-based sex, that's just dandy and I'm happy for ya. But one reason most couples let sex slide to the bottom of the "to do" list, right under "buy new sink plunger" and "get dog de-flead," is because they just don't have time at all. We have this belief that sex should be a fifteen-course banquet, lit with candles and surrounded by string quartets, and anything less seems like cheating. Well it's not. An orgasm is an orgasm, whether you arrived there after a five-hour car drive or by supersonic jet, so it's a

TIP

It sounds obvious but it isn't—if you're going to tease him, or he's going to tease you, you really should follow through. Whispering "when we get home I'm going to give you the best blow job you've ever had," then bottling out and falling asleep is just mean. And if he promises a three-act massage, sighing, "Yeah, but I wasn't tired when I said it," it's far worse than backing out on any other kind of bet—particularly if you're offering it as a bargaining tool. To avoid this, certain sex shops offer "gift vouchers" for sexual services, whereby you fill one in, give it to him, and it has to be cashed shortly after being produced. It's only fair.

If sex simply isn't happening because you're both too busy, and you can't even coordinate your schedules to ensure you're both in the same place at the same time, then you need to make a plan to have sex once a month. Once a month hardly sounds worth bothering with, but it's better than none a month—and quality in this situation is far more vital than quantity. Use it or lose it is also a truism when it comes to sex drive—so if you commit to at least one session a month it keeps you turning over.

shame that quickies are so underrated. Women always think that quickies exist simply for the pleasure of men, that all they involve is her hitching her skirt up and him going "uh-uh-uh-thanks," but they're wrong. Quickies can be equally appealing to both sexes because there's something deeply erotic about ignoring foreplay convention and heading straight for a good hard fuck. You don't have to take your clothes off to have a good time. Leaving things on just adds to the urgency and excitement. The best quickie is unexpected—when he's just got in from work, say, pin him against the wall and relieve him of his pants, then let him take you from behind. Or after a dinner party, sweep the leftovers to one side and do it on the kitchen table. You can even sneak around the back of a nightclub and do it under the fire escape, but you may well be interrupted by various drug dealers and their sniggering clientele, so go easy. A great time for a quickie is on your lunch hour—if you have time to sneak back home. Or if you're lucky enough to be having sex with a colleague, try the supply closet at work.

Quickies are a great way of showing each other that you still want each other and desire each other passionately—and even if you don't, the good news is you can invoke those feelings by going along with the idea and seeing what happens.

If he can't make you come in such a short space of time, just whip out your vibrator and hold it against your clitoris while he penetrates you—that should do the trick if nothing else does. And because an orgasm is good for you—it's relaxing, gets all the blood galloping around your body and fills you with giggly well-being—you can return to work after your lunchtime liaison entirely refreshed and happy. You don't get that from window shopping.

noise

Long-term sex does partially rely on remembering to demonstrate that you still like each other. So even if you're coming violently on a regular basis, if you simply lie there while he goes through the familiar old routine and then emit a little whimper at the end of it, he may very well start feeling that he isn't quite the god of love you once thought he was. So his performance will suffer accordingly, and he

TIP

Make a rule that he can't initiate sex for two weeks—which puts just enough pressure on you to do it yourself. Men get sick of always being the ones to risk rejection—it hurts, baby—so it's lovely for him to feel that he is wanted after all. It doesn't take much—just once in a while, make the first move with a kiss. Or given that most men like the direct approach, simply reach out and touch somebody by grabbing his penis under the bedsheets. Or on the plane if you're feeling particularly frisky.

Men love to hear that you're appreciating their moves in bed—in fact, a survey found that 80% like noisy sex, and the other 20% probably live with their parents. If you lie there in deadly silence, he won't know whether you're loving every second or mentally doing the bills. So even if it doesn't come naturally, make a noise anyway—just begin with a little gasp or groan; you don't need to have hysterics to begin with. Of course, as you get used to expressing yourself, hysterics may come naturally. If so, watch out for the neighbors. Thin walls are your worst enemy.

won't try as hard. So you'll be even less appreciative … and the same goes for him, too.

Yet it's so easy to raise your passion levels, and consequently his, without actually having an affair, or even pretending you're in a porno. All you have to do is make more noise. Yes, it's a little embarrassing, that can't be denied. But come on, a few groans and gasps are all that's needed to make him feel like King Dong, and you—once you've got over feeling silly—will be much more in touch with what you're feeling because you're reacting to every change of sensation, instead of just letting it happen.

He should also be vocal in his appreciation of whatever you're doing. Nobody wants a screamer—how many hotels have you stayed in, cursing the idiots in the next room who seem to think sex is supposed to be a five-act German opera? Nevertheless, totally silent sex is just as unnerving—so moan and whimper all you like, and encourage him to do the same.

> **TIP**
>
> If both of you are comfortable with the idea of writing, then take turns to write an erotic story for each other to read. You can make it as pornographic or romantic as you like, depending on what style turns you on. The chances are yours will be all "Desmond slipped the silken straps of Sophia's nightdress from her alabaster shoulders," and his will say, "'Put it in me,' groaned Angel, 'I'm still wet from fucking Venusia all night, and now I want your hot tool.'"

photo-me

Sound is one thing, accompanying visuals are quite another—and there are plenty of people who'd rather have their toenails removed with rusty pliers than commit their naked bodies to film. If you are one of them, don't agree to photos or video because you will automatically hate what you look like and spend the rest of the evening/week/year arguing about why you should have plastic surgery immediately, which really is not a basis for seductive conversation. Again, if you are someone who is a fundamental worrier, you will be instantly convinced that once these photos exist your mother will stumble upon them, or that you'll die prematurely and they'll be auctioned among your personal effects and all your friends and colleagues will come weeping to the auction, only to see "Lot 224, Miscellaneous Photographs" flashed up on a giant projector screen. Or if you've got kids, that their innocence will be destroyed as they ask, "Mommy, why is daddy hurting you in the picture?" Or … anyway, you get the point. So only do this if you don't hate your body, are reasonably confident that you know a decent hiding place, and trust that your partner won't dump you and post them on the internet (which is actually the most realistic possibility).

If you are, however, you should definitely consider the photo angle on sex. Light yourself well (soft but direct, so you don't get weird shadows that make you look like Ozzy Osbourne) and sit in the right position—sitting, your arms behind you so your breasts are thrust forward, stomach in, shot three-quarters on, makes everyone look good, as does lying on your side like the famous painting, *The Rokeby Venus*, because your waist automatically goes in and your legs are together, disguising less-than-perfect thighs. If he wants to pose, try sitting up, playing with his penis, or even standing up.

The best way to feature both of you is to video yourselves—you need to position a tripod at the end of the bed, focus the camera so the whole bed is in the shot, and then turn it on and make sure you stay roughly within view. After all, an entire tape of your joined calves and feet will not make for riveting viewing. You can get PC programs that will let you edit the tape, if it's digital, and add music and even sub-

---

TIP

Get yourself a Polaroid camera and have fun taking pictures of yourself in provocative poses—a picture of your breasts, or even genitals, can be enough to plummet him immediately into sexual mode—well, with most men just walking down the street can do that, but still. If you want to take a risk—and who doesn't, frankly?—then tuck one into his jacket pocket for him to find while he's away from you ... but perhaps you'd better leave a message telling him to do that when he's alone. Unless you want all his colleagues getting a good look at your Brazilian wax.

titles (well, you might want to pretend it's a French art-house movie—"Veronique! It's my father, he has arrived prematurely from Paris!" "Jean-Paul! I am also sleeping with your sister! Let's have a pastis," et cetera). Alternatively, you may just want to watch the basic tape and enjoy an actual porno starring yourselves. It's a lot more exciting than an actual porno starring large bleached bimbos—but make sure you label the tape carefully—you really don't want to give your friends an extra special treat when they come over to watch *Lord of the Rings*.

Spicing up your love life is well worth the effort—it may seem a little contrived or embarrassing at first, but if you persist you'll forget that you were trying at all because you'll be enjoying what you're doing so much. I'm convinced there'd be less affairs if there was more spicing up. Admittedly, it won't stop you fantasizing about other people, but it may well stop you from doing anything about it.

5   sex toys

Some people believe that sex on its own should be enough, without the unnecessary addition of sex toys. All that vibrating, whizzing plastic in the bedroom? Not for me! Then they wonder why their sex lives are so dull and repetitive and why it takes them hours to come. The truth is, sex toys are a vitally useful tool in your armory—not only do they provide you with an instant sex life should you happen to be single for a while, they also boost your sex life with a partner to no end. They can offer you the kind of thrills that normally you'd need a third person to administer—and your partner will almost certainly be grateful that you're getting your jollies from a bit of silicone, rather than his best friend.

Sex toys have come a long way from their rather shaky beginnings—once they were sold as "personal massagers" and required more technical know-how to wield than an AK47. Now you can get pretty much any kind of sex toy that floats your personal boat, from revolving love-eggs to blow-up sheep.

All the same, the old, miserable days of sneaking into dirty-looking "Adults Only XXX" shops on sketchy streets and plucking up the courage to ask for a vibrator that only came in one size and style—terrifying pink plastic—are long gone. Sex toys have come out of the closet, and while they're still some ways off from being displayed on the coffee table, they are more than acceptable purchases for the modern woman—and man. The only trouble is there are so many types it'd be

> **TIP**
>
> Vibrators are not just useful for genital stimulation—they're invaluable for locating your erogenous zones as well. Set it to "low" and try it against your breasts, nipples, neck and inner thighs—in fact, try it anywhere that you suspect might be an erogenous zone and would like to check. It also works wonders for his balls. And don't ignore his nipples, either—as you will discover, they still respond to vibration.

impossible to try them all. If you still can't face going into a shop and asking a live assistant, even though they've seen it all before a hundred thousand times, you can order what you want over the internet. It will arrive in plain packaging and, trust me, the mailman will never know—unless you decide to give him a private showing.

sex toys for girls

Girls tend to do better when it comes to sex toys than men. That may be because sex toys for women are fun additions to a healthy sex life, or a handy way of having an orgasm when you're alone. For men, however, sex toys are often packaged as a weird substitute for a girl-friend—"so real!," "Wanda has an amazing 3-speed vagina," and so on—which, at the very least, is just creepy. If you've ever seen those odd-looking rubber butts with horrible synthetic hair coming out of plastic follicles I'm sure you understand where I'm coming from. Still, they probably make a lot of men very happy, so it's best to leave them to their world of fun with Blowup Bambi and concentrate on what sex toys can do for girls.

vibrators

There are thousands of different types of vibrators—but they all aim to do the same thing: stimulate your clitoris and vagina and smooth the path to an orgasm. Some are so powerful they can make you come in seconds, others offer a more gentle journey via a faint tingling sensation that culminates in a few rhythmic contractions of the vagina, rather than the screaming, breathless helter-skelter that the really big hitters hope to give you. It's a nice idea to keep different types for different occasions, although as sex toys get more sophisticated they offer different attachments and speeds in the same model. This is getting a little like buying motorcycles, and about as confusing, so let's get back to basics. Vibrators come either electricity-powered or battery-powered. If they require lots of whizzing, buzzing attachments, they may have a battery pack attached to them, or the battery might be one of the little disc-shaped integral ones. With cheaper models the battery often fails to fit properly, which means you'll be seconds away from the biggest orgasm of your life, when there's a little "clunk" and you

---

TIP

If he's using a vibrator on you—or you are on his ass—it really helps to have some vocal guidance. Without any nerves it's almost impossible for him to tell whether he's pushing too fast, or too hard—so if you can say "that's perfect … bit further … stop there," it will save him a lot of worry, trying to interpret whether your sharp intakes of breath meant "oh, god, no!" or just "oh yes! Yes!" And, of course, he should extend a similar courtesy to you.

---

realize it's slipped sideways and the whole thing's just ground to a halt. The electric ones are safer—but you do need to plug them in, obviously, and on the down side, they really aren't very quiet.

Vibrators come in all manner of sizes and shapes, ranging from the discreet handbag-friendly mini-dildo kind to the enormous, throbbing, 14-inch sort that should probably only be used in the dressing rooms of heavy metal bands by trashed groupies. For everyone else they're just too much to deal with. Certain men, in particular, get horribly insecure when confronted with giant vibrators and begin to compare themselves unfavorably with their plastic rivals. Reassure him all you like, but if you're unpacking Wayne the 12-inch Wonder-wand for the third time this week, he may have reason to be concerned. So, don't start being unfaithful to him with your vibrator to the extent that you actually prefer it.

You can get vibrators that are disguised as anything—from religious artifacts (one for all you lapsed Catholics out there) to giant corncobs to lipstick tubes. Most of them, however, do the same thing—which is to provide something to put inside your vagina that resem-

TIP

It is possible to buy sex toys that exist mainly to encourage you to tighten your vaginal muscles. Obviously, should your partner buy you these, you must immediately stuff them up a different hole altogether (belonging to him). However, if it's your decision, then the tension required to hold them in place ensures that your PC muscles get a continual workout. Of course, there's always the worry that you'll forget and they'll drop out mid-subway ride. Which would be bad.

bles a penis (lesbians often buy "goddess"-shaped vibrators to avoid this, but at the end of the day, they just resemble a penis with bad hair) and something to tickle your clitoris, which can be a separate attachment, or part of the wand itself, which you hold against yourself. Some prefer to run them up and down while they vibrate, others to hold them in the most sensitive place and wait for nirvana. Some even treat them like sports cars, flicking between speeds like Jeff Gordon flicks between gears.

Most vibrators are straight, but some are bendy, designed to reach the G-spot—and they probably do have a better chance of doing that than fingers. Natural Contours (designed by Candida Royalle) are a range that are shaped to fit your shape, and actually don't look like penises—they're curvy, come in different lengths, and nestle beautifully against your pubic mound.

The best-known vibrator is probably the Rabbit. It's G-spot friendly, with a rotating section full of little beads in the middle, and rabbit "ears" to tickle your clitoris with. It's also a huge seller, having been featured on "Sex & The City"—and if it was good enough for Samantha ....

duotone balls

Duotone balls are, in certain people's opinions—alright, that might just be mine—somewhat overrated. They are two little prickly spheres made of silicone, or the like, which are inserted into your vagina. Once there, they're supposed to roll about, stimulating as they go. But in truth, not only is it like trying to get a hedgehog's tampon up there, if you push them too far you can't feel a thing—as is with tampons—and if you don't, it feels like they're about to fall out. Again, like tam-

TIP

It is possible to buy sex toys such as the Butterfly with a remote-control attachment. So for a night out with a much more entertaining difference, stick the vibrating bit in your underwear, give him the controls, and enjoy. Actually, the difference could be the screaming fight you have when you hand him the controls and he turns the buzzer off just as you're about to come. That aside, as long as you know how to disguise the fact that you're turned on (and if you ever entertained boys at your parents' house, you probably do), go ahead.

pons. If you do manage to get them balanced somewhere acceptable, who knows, you might be beside yourself with excitement in no time—but I kind of doubt it.

butterfly

This is much more useful—the Butterfly (though it goes under various other names) is a little vibrating disc that hooks over your hips almost like a jock strap. The idea then is, you put your underwear on over it to hold it in place against your clitoris, and off you go—climaxing as you go about your domestic duties, or attend high-level business meetings, or what-have-you. It's a very sexy idea, but in practice it could be a bit of a nightmare—you really don't need to be all red and flushed as you enjoy Sunday dinner with your boyfriend's parents—unless, of course, his Dad's really that attractive.

waterproof

Waterproof vibrators are ideal for the active woman caught in a rainstorm who wants an orgasm to take her mind off the weather ... or then again, they may simply be suitable for use in the bath and shower. This is a great idea, since for a lot of women the bathroom's the only place they're likely to get enough peace and quiet to masturbate—particularly if you live in a shared house, or have kids. You can purchase ones that are cunningly disguised to look like a sponge—put it between your legs in the bath or shower and away you go; all the fun of an orgasm, none of the electrocution. In fact, be careful—make sure it definitely is waterproof before you go ahead and jump in with it. Otherwise, what an embarrassing way to go.

clit stimulators

The finger tickler is a thoroughly ingenious little device. It just looks like a baby splint—alright, it's not that sexy, but still … and it straps on to your finger—or his—which is then, of course, placed against the clitoris. So you get free access to your vagina, and lots of clitoral stimulation without the unwieldy interference of a big dildo getting in the way.

dildos

And speaking of dildos … they are just penis-shaped objects used in place of an actual penis. They're handy for anal penetration while he's inside you, or for using if his penis is having an off day, or he's just come three times and is exhausted. The double-ended ones are for double penetration. Niiice!

condoms

Condoms are not, strictly speaking, a sex toy, admittedly. But they do come in all kinds of guises, which include French Ticklers. Possibly not a phrase used in the last 50 years, still, the condom with an added part—typically, a cockscomb or sea urchin–like piece made of latex—

TIP

For an inexpensive vibrator, you can't beat an electric toothbrush. Just make sure no one's planning on using it to clean their teeth later. Aside from that, though, it works on exactly the same principle, and should deliver a similar thrill when it vibrates against your clitoris. If you like a little erotic abrasion, you can hold the bristles against yourself—but if, like most people, you think that sounds less fun than a bikini wax, just press the back of the head against your clitoris, an instruction that works well for oral sex, too.

are still available. The idea being that they reach the parts that penises cannot reach (that damned G-spot again) and stimulate it to no end. This is based on the premise that he can actually roll on a condom that features a novelty penguin balancing on the tip without collapsing in hysterics. A better bet, perhaps, are ribbed condoms, which actually are quite useful when it comes to creating friction—the basis of all sexual excitement. If you're very wet, his penis can go in so smoothly it's barely noticeable—but a ribbed condom slows the process down, and makes sure you feel him moving. Worth buying a pack, and much cheaper than plastic surgery.

diy

You can, of course, avoid purchasing any sex toys whatsoever and make do with whatever you have in your house. Clothes pins for nipple clamps—be advised, plastic ones are less painful—or even paper clips, should you be suddenly overcome with an urge for a nipple clamp while at the office.

For vibrators, the economy version is the electric toothbrush. Small, discreet and you can easily get it through customs without dying of embarrassment. You can even set your cell phone to "vibrate," and get all your friends to ring you up. But that's not the best idea. Dildos are easier—and there's always cucumbers, bananas, eggplants (ow!), carrots, corn on the cob … in fact, why are so many vegetables penis-shaped? There's a question.

Some women, I'm told, even use rounded-end deodorant bottles. But that's not very safe—and so embarrassing if it gets lodged up there.

sex toys for him

Sex toys for men are not quite as varied and interesting as those aimed at women. Maybe that's because men are less likely to need help orgasming. Or maybe they just have less orifices to put things in. Well … they definitely do. Still, there are certain devices that can change a dull night into a fantastic one with the simple aid of a battery—or even just a bit of plastic.

cock rings

These are bendy little bits of plastic that fit around the base of his penis. The idea is that they retain his erection, and ensure that the maximum amount of blood fills it, keeping it hard and stiff. This increases the sensitivity for him, but is even better for you. Some cock rings even have attachments that rub your clitoris as he thrusts. In fact, this is just as much a sex toy for you as it is for him … still, who's complaining?

vibrators

Vibrators can do wonders for men, once they get over their occasional fears that using them is somehow girly. He should switch it to the strongest speed and hold it against his penis—hey presto, instant erection—or put it on a lower setting and caress his balls with it. He can even push it into his anus, where it will do marvelous things by stimulating his prostate gland. The best kind of vibrator for a man is a fairly simply dildo-shaped or Natural Contours one, which you can trail over the tip of his penis, or hold alongside the shaft, splint-like, till he's all big and strong again. If you're feeling too lazy to give a hand job, it's a great way of turning him on, and you can use it while you give him a blow job, as long as you don't mind your mouth going all weird and tingly. You can get cock rings that vibrate, but that may feel a little too much like being a food-processor for most men, and, unless he has a deep urge to stick his penis into cake mix, perhaps it's best avoided.

anal beads

Rather like a rosary in appearance, anal beads do what they say on the container—they're beads, and they go up his ass. The idea is that you push them up there, leave a little thread hanging out, and just as he's about to come, you pull them out with a theatrical flourish and give him a titanic orgasm of epic proportions. Should you attempt this, you will, of course, be using lubrication—and you will not shout, "Oh my god, I just thought, they might have poo on them!" at the crucial moment. Not unless you want to give him sexual hang-ups for the rest of his life. You can even get rigid ones, which do much the same thing—and if you're of a craft-making disposition, you can even make your own! But make sure they're tightly tied on, you really don't want to be explaining to the nurse why he's got half a Guatemalan bracelet up his ass.

blow up!

Let's just clarify now, we're only including blow-up dolls for the sake of thoroughness … it's extremely unlikely that he'll be attempting to introduce one into your love-making sessions. However realistic (and these days, the expensive ones are freakishly like having sex with a busty starlet, even down to the plastic content and conversational ability), if he does suggest that Silicone Suzy joins you in the boudoir, you're at full liberty to stick a pin in her thigh and watch her deflate.

sex gloves

These are simply gloves with different textures on the fingers—and again, if you were feeling a bit arts-and-crafty, you could make your own. They may have one finger fur, one leather, one lace, one rubber … you get the idea. So you just try out each one on his skin and see which produces the best effect. Hopefully not fur, or you'll be out trapping bears to turn him on before you know it. Leather's always a good bet—so maybe Dad's driving gloves could be put to a whole new purpose ….

mints

Sex shops sell all kinds of liquids that you're supposed to paste on and lick off—"penis growing lotion," "booby drops," you know the kind of thing. And they're weirdly flavored like stale licorice, despite the flavor they claim to be. However, you can enjoy a much more profound effect simply with an extra-strong mint. Just suck one for a while, and then lick and suck his penis. The effect will be instant—not quite pain, but enough stimulation to make all his nerve endings start firing madly. If it hurts, alternate with mouthfuls of water. Don't get carried away and rub the mint directly onto his skin—unless, of course, you really, really hate him.

diy

There are, once again, a variety of household objects that lend themselves to pleasing his penis to no end. Fruit and vegetables aren't quite as perfect as they are for you. After all, not many are vagina-shaped. So your best bet is to eat fruit off his penis (see Chapter 4 for details) and save the vegetables for anal penetration if that's what he likes.

You can also use items that give him new sensations—feathers trailed along his penis and used to tickle his balls will provide a fantastic thrill for him, and he can always return the favor on your inner thighs. You can use a feather duster if you wish, but it's a bit much for some tastes. A simple ostrich feather (what do you mean you don't have any lying around?) should work.

There are certain things you can wrap around his penis when you're giving him a hand job that will ensure a spectacular orgasm—chief among these is a pearl necklace. As well as being slang for him coming all over your breasts, the real thing can produce sensations that your hand just isn't capable of giving him.

Just wrap your string of pearls—and of course fake ones are just as good—around his penis as many times as they'll go, then put your hand over them and proceed with a normal hand job. The feeling of the little bumps rubbing all over his penis is highly erotic—but if you don't want him to ejaculate all over Granny's pearls, make sure you whip them away in plenty of time.

You can try the same effect with silk scarves, wooden beads, pieces of fun fur, chip bags … actually, maybe not chip bags. But anything else painless and sexy to the touch is worth a try.

sex toys during sex

So far, the whole idea has revolved around taking turns: you do something, then he does something to you. But certain sex toys come into their own during sex itself, and you can both share them. The best way is to hold a vibrator in between you during sex, so it's pressing on your clitoris and his balls at the same time. Alternatively, you can hold it against his balls and anus while he thrusts into you, or lie so it's angled at your own anus—or inside it—while he's inside your vagina. Vibrators can also be rubbed across your breasts, or his nipples—in fact, the only thing not worth doing with one is attempting to kiss it.

games & props

Playing sexual games is a great way to introduce a little more fun into your sex life without joining a swingers' group. They are particularly good for slightly inhibited people, since the games' rules dictate what you have to do. As long as you go along with the rules, you have no say in the matter, which frees you up nicely to be as outrageous as you want.

strip poker … and the rest

Strip games are the perfect way to begin a sex session. Especially with someone you'd like to have sex with but are too shy to actually make a move on. Strip poker is only one version—and if you're not sure of the rules, the beauty of this game is that the strip part can be adapted to almost any other competitive game. Strip Monopoly might take a really long time, though. Ideally, what you want is a game that will result in great, sweeping reversals of fortune, allowing forfeits and tension to come in as well. Something like 21, or blackjack, are good card games to try—that way it's all in the hands of fate rather than on your skill.

If you find the clothes are coming off too fast, and you want to prolong the simmering sexual tension, then simply add forfeits to the mix—sexual ones, of course. He might have to lick your nipples for one minute, or you might have to masturbate in front of him—anything to crank up the desire between you without actually fulfilling it. And the game lasts as long as you can bear it to.

blindman's buff

You take turns to be blindfolded. Whoever can see conceals a small item somewhere about their naked body, and the blindfoldee has to locate it. The amusing twist on this one is, that he or she can only search with their mouth, so kissing, licking and nibbling are all allowed; touching is not. It goes without saying that the hider will become increasingly sophisticated when it comes to where the item is hidden—although it does count as cheating to keep moving it. Suggested items are a Hershey's Kiss, or a raspberry—nothing that can be choked on, though. And when it's found, you swap roles. Or rip off the blindfold and make mad, passionate love—whichever comes first.

porn charades

This is extremely simple, yet strangely effective. All you have to do is act out whatever you'd like to have done to you without actually speaking. So if you want to be taken from behind, you simply adopt the doggy position, and thrust your butt in the air. But it's more complicated if you also want him to caress your clitoris at the same time with a vibrator. And if he wants to stand in front of a mirror watching you masturbate, how's he going to get that across without props ...? Play it naked, and when anyone guesses correctly, they get to do it for real. If they don't, it's the other player's turn. A word of warning, though—it's not one for family gatherings.

porno snap

Again, simple—you simply rent a porno, and every time the actors do something, you do it, too. It helps not to rent one about a gang bang though, unless you have a really strong relationship. Ideal ones feature hilariously unattractive models so neither of you gets jealous. You just keep an eye on what's happening, and follow the leaders on screen. At the very least, it should give you an entertaining sexual workout. And if you see her deep-throating him and wonder what her secret is? Don't worry, it's just camera trickery. It doesn't really happen unless you're a sword-swallower, and that is not a game I'd recommend.

fantasy and roleplay

Fantasy deserves a whole book to itself—as Nancy Friday proved with her series featuring women's and men's deepest erotic thoughts. Your fantasies are your business, and there's no law that says you have to share them with your partner—besides, he may not want to know your most private thoughts about zoo keepers and such. And you may not really wish to delve too thoroughly into his issues with his ex-girlfriend and a jar of jam. However, shared fantasies are an entirely different kettle of fish (though if he's fantasizing about one, stop right there, you may not want to know).

If you have the courage to tell each other what turns you on, you're opening up a whole new chapter of your shared sexuality, which can unleash feelings you never knew you had and clear the way for some fantastic experiences. Because once you've opened up and made sure he isn't reeling in horror, you can enact your fantasies in real life. That's "enact," notice, not "live out"—which is an entirely different thing. Pretending to be a hooker is a long way from standing on the interstate with no undies on, eyeing truck drivers.

And pretending he's a wicked principal and you're a naughty schoolgirl is a very long way from the dreadful court case that would ensue should he try it for real.

When it comes to discussing your fantasies, particularly those you'd like to act out, it pays to go easy at first—there's nothing worse than one's partner breathing "you what?" in disgust and horror before flinging back the comforter and going to cry in the bathroom. So leave out all references to any of his friends or family members you've always found attractive, never mention exes, and go easy on the whole Brad Pitt thing, especially if he looks nothing like him whatsoever.

Suitable fantasies for sharing will generally include a role for each other—so if you'd like to be a lap dancer let him be the paying customer, or if you fancy being a sassy businesswoman, allow him to be the nervous interviewee for the position of your assistant. The same goes for him—if he'd like to be the Lord of the Manor, you can be the housemaid, or the vinyl-clad dominatrix to his trembling love-slave. It's vital that you're both happy with the roles you're assigned, and you aren't both striving for power at the expense of the game—"No! I'm the Roman Emperor! You're just a slave!" "Fuck off! I thought of it in the first place!" doesn't make for great sex.

Once you've decided on your scenario, however, you'll need to get some props together to help you make the scene vaguely convincing. Look, it doesn't need to be all that convincing, you just have to make it faintly believable for the duration of foreplay and sex—calm down, no one's going to be asking the director about their motivation or anything.

Useful props to have are: a cape (works for evil headmasters, superheroes, vampires, Florence Nightingale and dominatrixes), very sexy high heels (works for everything, but particularly hookers and lap dancers), glasses (works for the business interview because you can remove them from each other at the crucial moment), suits (good for business, again—also, in his case, a high-class escort's customer), pearls (see above, also ideal for Lady Chatterley types), an apron and white hat (good for nurses and maids), and a peaked cap (chauffeurs, policemen).

Of course you can supplement your dressing-up box with whatever else you want: firemen's helmets, lady-in-distress nighties … whatever suits your particular fantasies—even a rubber gimp mask and a pair of marabou-trimmed slippers.

erotica

Sex toys, games and props can all be helped along by a little sprinkle of one final thing—no, not drugs, you at the back—erotica, which includes books, films and magazines. Indeed, you may call it porn if you wish, but we're not necessarily talking about hardcore action.

Books such as the *Herotica* series aimed at women—but almost certainly read by men—are perfect erotica in that they contain a storyline and characters who aren't simply vessels for sperm—but at the same time they do spend most of their lives fucking in a variety of interesting and challenging new ways. The books are perfect for you to read before he arrives in bed—thus bringing you to the level of sexual arousal that men tend to simmer at most of the time—or for you to read to each other.

Magazines, too, have their place—in your house that might be "on a fire," but bear with me. The market has expanded in a bid to fight the encroaching porn provision of the internet, and the newer magazines are aiming themselves at couples, with literate writing and photo shoots of gorgeous people in interesting positions rather than the usual dimwit teen in a spread-eagle pose, which may not, understandably, appeal. Erotica allows you to explore the sides of your sexuality you've kept under wraps—your secret fantasies about women, say, or his occasional thoughts about group sex—and brings it into the open in a non-threatening way.

Pornos, too, are worth considering as an erotic tool. Nowadays, it is possible to buy the kind that are made with women in mind, which may actually feature some kind of plot, and a heroine who sometimes has fully formed thoughts before she opens her legs. If all that sounds way too scary and hardcore, consider erotic books— Anais Nin, Erica Jong, even D.H. Lawrence have all written literature that has been, in its day, considered obscene. Now, however, they're considered classics, and you could happily read them on the subway. Or, better still, in bed.

6 adventurous sex

Adventurous sex suggests you're doing it on some mosquito-infested bank somewhere in Borneo, or up K2 with only a sleeping bag between you and certain death. However, you can have wildly adventurous sex without going farther than the bedroom—and besides, sex on K2 is incredibly dull. I know, I've tried it. (Obviously, this is a lie.)

Adventurous sex is all about pushing the boundaries, trying things you've never done before—and possibly things you wouldn't tell your friends, should they ask. Well, you've got to have some secrets, don't you? We're not talking about sketchy, risky, picking-up-strangers sex—you go right ahead if you like that, but I refuse to take the blame

---

TIP

Magazines always rave about the hot/cold blow job, which is, ultimately, just slightly painful and not that much fun, given that most versions seem to involve you taking alternate sucks of ice and chili. But if you simply sip on a chilled glass of white wine, and then nibble a bit of ginger, it'll be far less unpleasant—for both of you. And he'll still get the remarkable sensations of heat and cold on his penis. He can return the favor, but not quite as hot and not quite as cold—you're more sensitive, see?

---

when it turns out he was an escaped convict/crazy/emotionally stunted. We are, however, talking about sketchy, risqué, picking-up-your-partner-and-whirling-him-over-your-head sex.

Anything you can think of that two (or more) people can do sexually without getting arrested counts as adventurous sex. At the very least, it probably involves leaving the lights on.

anal sex

Anal sex can result in some stunning orgasms and sensations. And it's not the once-in-a-lifetime experiment it used to be—a Playboy survey reveals that 47% of men and 67% of women have tried anal intercourse … which begs the question, who or what were the extra 20% of women having it with? Looks like somebody's lying … or else they're lesbians and counting penetration with dildos as intercourse, or there's a few men out there having anal sex with lots of different women. Let's hope they're using condoms. Interestingly, the biggest increase in sex toys is in anal toy sales, so if everybody's at it, surely it pays to know exactly what's worth bothering with.

Anal sex is every man's fantasy. Well, not strictly every man—probably just 99.9% and the .1% are scared it'll make them gay. They'd like to if they weren't so uptight …. Men love it, you see, because not only is it forbidden, and therefore thoroughly dirty—in the best sense

---

TIP

If you're going to have anal sex, bear in mind that while it's not dangerous, my best advice is to limit it to once every few weeks—and if you can't sit down the next day, that's probably more than enough.

TIP

When you're already stimulated, you're more relaxed, so it's easier for him to slide a finger into your anus. It still helps to use lubrication, though, and go slowly. If he pushes a finger in while he's got another in your vagina, the combined pressure can be much more stimulating than just anal penetration by itself. Moving his fingers with a slow in-and-out rhythm should provide an exciting sensation around your G-spot, too.

of the word—it's also a fantastically tight fit because the anus is not meant to accommodate a baby, it's only meant to accommodate ... well, yes, anyway. So it's a lot smaller, has no natural lubrication, and basically offers the most fantastic, friction-packed experience on a man's penis that he could wish for without forking out for a team of highly trained call boys with the internal muscle control of cocaine traffickers. So no wonder he likes it.

As for women, some absolutely love it because of its naughty nature, and the hard stimulating effect on their vaginas. If you are going to give your partner the chance to fulfill this particular lifetime ambition, there's a few things you should know first. Most importantly, whatever you believe about your bowels prolapsing, it's not true. You'd have to be having a hell of a lot of anal sex, with a hell of a lot of big dicks, for that to even be an option. And assuming you're not, have no fear, your anus will spring back into its normal tiny shape soon afterwards. So if that's the kind of thing you spend a lot of time worrying about, rest assured.

Secondly, if you are going to do it, you need to be very well lubricated around there. It will really hurt if you try it from a standing start, believe me. A generous helping of KY should do, unless you're so wildly aroused you can generate enough yourself to do the job—but even so, on this occasion, the wetter the better. Beforehand, he should have made sure to spend enough time on foreplay to relax you entirely—it's no good assuming the position and hissing, "Come on, get it over with," through gritted teeth. Well, you can, but that may kill the atmosphere.

He should also make sure to use a condom—the skin of the anus is not made for friction and tears very easily, so any diseases can gallop right into your bloodstream and wreak havoc. It's also not the most sterile environment for him to be sticking his penis in, either—so you may as well err on the side of caution with this one. The best position for anal sex—and I'm sure your Mother will already have told you this—is doggy style. But don't thrust your butt as high as you would with ordinary doggy—you really don't want penetration that deep, because until you're used to it, it will be a squeeze at best and agonizing at worst. He must push very gently—regardless of how excited he is—until the tip has penetrated your anus. If you find you've clenched up

---

TIP

If you feel compelled to rim—where you lick each other's butts, like little doggies—the only thing that's really important is to be clean because this region is a breeding ground for odd bacteria, which is fine when butt-bound but not so good in your mouth. It's a good idea to keep a pack of baby wipes by the bed so you can just whisk it over your genitals should the urge to lick where the sun don't shine overtakes you. And if you can overcome your natural inhibitions, it can feel fantastic, so it's definitely worth the price of a wipe.

Reassuringly, anal sex toys all have a little flange, which stops them from disappearing up inside, and prevents emergency room staff from being harassed nightly by herds of humiliated men, all with plastic dildos wedged up their butts. So if you want specific toys for anal penetration, make sure you get the ones that state what they're for and have taken this into account in their design. It's a lot easier for stuff to disappear up asses than up vaginas—hence the number of hilarious nurses' tales, about light bulbs, cucumbers, vacuums … and as far as I know, vacuums don't come with a flange. You can also buy a butt plug—a charmingly romantic name, I'm sure you'll agree—that inserts into the anus. Some actually vibrate, and the inflating sort expands to twice its original size and stimulates the male G-spot.

with nerves, don't panic, just allow him to use his fingers to very gently massage and stretch the hole slightly. He can insert one finger first, followed by two—if he gets carried away and keeps going until he's inserting whole cucumbers, though, that's the time to ask questions.

Once he's able to get it in—and if he is the proud owner of a really, really big penis, he may have to accept that he never will, since this is the one time having a small one is a positive advantage—he should go slooooowly. Just push it a couple of inches in, and almost come out again. If at this point, you are shouting "ooow!" then perhaps it's not going to happen tonight. If you're merely thinking "hmm, what a bizarre and strangely exciting feeling," then you may go right ahead. If you can take it, he can thrust gently in as far as feels comfortable—not for him, he's having a whale of a time—for you. The problem will come when he's well on the way to an orgasm and is tempted suddenly to speed up dramatically and thrust in a downright reckless fashion, which may well translate into downright painful. So he must be constantly vigilant that he isn't getting carried away and hurting you. Of course, there's a chance that you too may be getting carried away and shouting "go, go, go!" in which case go ahead. But don't blame me when you can't sit down tomorrow.

You can have anal sex in any position—but the other one that works well is you bending over the table, since it provides easy access to the correct hole for him, and gives you something to brace yourself against. Missionary position is useless for anal sex, don't even attempt it. But if you do the table thing, don't tell the relatives what you were doing on it last night when they arrive for Sunday lunch. And you can go on top—but it's hard to get it in from that angle, so don't be surprised if it all ends in collapse.

Just to be sensible for a moment, he shouldn't penetrate your vagina after he's been in your anus because that's a very handy way to transfer tons of bacteria that you really don't want in there. Other than that, go ahead. He can penetrate you with a dildo while you have anal sex if that appeals, or you can penetrate him with a dildo, he can

---

TIP

Everyone has a different threshold for pain, but generally, women can take more pain than men. This is worth remembering whatever you're doing, but particularly relevant when it comes to S&M. What feels like a stimulating slap to you can be an agonizing blow to him—so if you are wielding the cane, you need to make sure you're being careful, and letting him set the pace.

If you're going to spank each other with a cane, choose it with care—the last thing you want are great red welts all over your ass. Half the eroticism, too, is in the swishing motion—hearing it whisk through the air builds the excitement before it strikes, and a great big wooden stick won't do that—but a small, bendy one will. Practice first with a bamboo garden stake, and based on how much pain you find a turn-on—if any—buy a cane that's thicker or thinner, accordingly.

have his fingers inside you at the same time as he's penetrating your anus ... oh, my, the possibilities are endless.

Of course, the irony is, his anus features a prostate gland, which makes anal penetration an absolute party in the park for him. You, however, have no prostate. Still, life's a funny thing, eh? For him, anal penetration will usually be with fingers. You need to insert a very well-lubricated finger about an inch and a half, to a point where you'll feel two sphincter muscles against the side when you press—the gland you're looking for is another couple of inches in, on the front wall, and when touched feels sensational.

sado masochism

Sadism is named after the Marquis de Sade, who enjoyed inflicting pain. And Masochism is named after Baron Sacher-Masoch, who enjoyed receiving it. Obviously, the two would have been a perfect pairing, but sadly they never met. Most couples, however, who favor a little S&M activity tend to take the opposing roles—it's rare to find serious S&M-ers who take turns because when giving or receiving

TIP

If dressing up in tight rubber appeals, it pays to know that getting into it is like struggling into a full-body condom. That is, difficult and sometimes painful. But a way of making it easier to slide on without catching yourself painfully is with liberal applications of talcum powder, which smooths over all your lumps and bumps beautifully. Getting out of it, however is a different matter—and unless you want to crush his "mystery woman" fantasy totally, you might want to do this in private.

pain or control forms a large part of somebody's sexuality, it tends to stay in a certain direction. For those who are merely playing, though, it's entirely possible to swap roles around and try personas on for size.

One of you is dominant, one submissive. It isn't necessarily about inflicting actual pain on your partner—S&M can be as mild as being blindfolded and doing his or her bidding. But it can be as strong as being whipped, hung from a harness, or strapped and handcuffed, being beaten with a cat o' nine tails. Exploring deeply into the world of S&M requires a great deal of trust in each other, and total understanding of what is and isn't too dangerous to experiment with. And as this is not the S&M handbook, for our purposes we'll assume you don't have a huge fetish, and that you'd simply like a bit of leather-based love-life spicing.

dressing the part

The easiest way to start your journey into the world of pain and pleasure (or, at least, fluffy handcuffs) is with the dress code. S&M-ers like leather, rubber and vinyl, all fabrics that mold to the body, feel like skin, only with a harder edge, and carry a suggestion of restraint—

most garments either expose a lot of flesh, or are extremely tight and figure-revealing, with bondage straps, studs and shiny parts. The look is, of course, highly sexy on women—most men take one look and think "Michelle Pfeiffer. Catwoman. Yesss!" even if you look more like Tina Turner in *Mad Max*. On men, however, it's slightly less than hot, unless he gets it absolutely right—and studded vinyl speedos don't work for many men, it has to be said. Wait, make that "any." He might just about get away with leather pants and motorcycle boots— though he may only attain "hairdresser out clubbing"—and a studded belt, a dog collar and leather gloves might be acceptable, too. The full rubber gimp-mask look, however, is probably best saved for the hardcore fan. A long, black leather coat makes any man look like Steve McQueen, and a few chains—particularly through his nipples— should complete the "S&M Lite" look.

For you, high heels are essential—ideally, shiny thigh-high boots covered in buckles. Sex shops sell vast ranges of leather, metal and stud-encrusted clothing, most of which has special holes for breasts and penises. So don't be shy.

TIP

When you're tying each other up, it's useful to use restraints you can actually undo afterward. Which is why anything with nylon in it is a really bad idea, and silk or cotton is fine. Using discarded stockings, then, while a dirtily attractive notion, is a disaster in reality because the lycra tightens to a flesh-choking grip, and the knots are impossible to undo. The best bet is silk scarves.

---

s&m accessories

If you're committed to the S&M thing, you'll need a few props—chief of which is handcuffs. Handcuffs are ideal for pinning you down so you can't wriggle away (as countless policemen have discovered over the years). They are, though, easy to use wrongly—and putting your hands behind your back and cuffing them is painful after only a couple of minutes, not to mention stupidly uncomfortable. You should have your wrists handcuffed to the headboard of the bed—or the nearest piece of heavy furniture. Your arms should be above your head, but not stretched so hard you're popping your shoulder joints out of place with every movement—make sure there's some bend in your elbows. You can get ankle, cuffs, too, to pin each leg to the end of the bed—all of which relies on your having some kind of old Victorian brass bed—so if you don't have one, you'd better sell your postless one and buy one, right?

There are even special sheets you can purchase with integral foot and wrist straps, but in all honesty they do make you look like something out of *One Flew Over the Cuckoo's Nest*, so don't invest in one

TIP

If you want to try bondage but handcuffs seem a bit hardcore, you can buy bondage tape from sex shops—like duct tape, but not nearly as hard to unpeel; it simply wraps around your ankles or wrists without causing pain, and can be pulled or snipped off when you've finished. You can use it as a gag, theoretically—but gagging can be a dangerous move, so go easy and don't wrap it around each other's heads six times or anything.

TIP

> You can get leather dog collars and leads to drag your sex-slave around behind you—and wear them to a private club (no, not the local Rotary Association, you fool) or simply play Master and Servant at home. If you do, though, be extra-vigilant about how much force you're using—power-games can tap into all sorts of buried emotions, and you don't want to be getting off on the fantasy only to turn around and find he's sobbing because of his unresolved issues. So go easy.

unless you have some Jack Nicholson/Nurse Ratched fantasy thing going on, OK?

You may also like to purchase a little whip, or a cat o' nine tails—which is a little whip with tiny leather strands coming out of it, and gives a softer swish to the buttocks. You don't have to whack the living crap out of your partner with it, just give him a tingly little slap on the butt. And a backhand stroke gives you a better angle for a smooth whip than a forward stroke, though you can alternate the two, back and forth, like an angry ping-pong player. There's a little whisk-y one you can buy, called The Devil's Hair Whip Black—it gives a sharp sensation without actually causing untold damage—so that's the kind of thing you should be investigating if you're really serious.

You can buy custom-made blindfolds, all lovely and leather—or you can just make do with his winter scarf if that seems a bit of a wild extravagance. Or compromise with a silk one.

Of course for the serious S&M-er, there's a vast range of equipment, from rubber coffins to tapes of white noise intended to disorient masochist love-slaves. But perhaps that end of the market will not be troubling you.

what to do

The association of pain with pleasure is a complex one, and while some find any kind of stimulation arousing, others may hate the sensation of experiencing pain during sex. The theory is that when you're aroused, you're filled with endorphins, which enable you to undergo stronger sensations than you'd normally withstand—but that doesn't mean you have to like having your ass spanked. And just in case you don't but your partner's lost in a world of flaring nostrils and cracking whips, those clever S&M people have come up with a code that means "stop."

In S&M games, "No" can mean all kinds of things. It can mean "Oh my god! Yes! Yes! No! I'm so excited!" Or it can mean "No! I'm pretending to be a virgin you're deflowering! Don't stop!" Or … well, it can mean all sorts of other things if you're role-playing. So to make sure that if your handcuffs are starting to chafe painfully, or your whipping isn't going according to plan, you use the traffic-light code

---

TIP

DIY S&M is a whole lot easier to sort out than the kind where you have to explain to a pimply teenage assistant exactly what you want to do with that rubber diving suit. And S&M props can be found around the house … try tight rubber dishwashing gloves for a different hand-job sensation, clothespins for nipple clamps (yes, you may look stupid, but think of the money you're saving), and a soft hairbrush for a little light spanking.

If you have a fantasy that you want to confess to your partner but you don't know how he'll react, find an erotic story that deals with the theme (and if you can't find one, OK, maybe you're a little creative ...) and leave it lying around the bathroom. Then later ask if he happened to see it and what he thought of it. If he says, "Oh my god, that's so perverted! Some people are beyond belief," then perhaps it's best left a private fantasy. But if he says, "Whoa, that's a bit of a turn-on," then you might just be in luck.

instead. If you want to stop, you say "Red!"—there's no other context you could use this word in, so he—or you—will immediately know what you mean. And if you're worried he might stop, you simply shout "Green!" for "go ahead with what you're doing." Presumably, if you quite like it but you don't want him to get completely carried away, you say "Yellow." Now there's passion!

blindfolding

When you're blindfolded, you are basically in the submissive role. You have no control over what's going on—and if you're tied up as well, you're about as powerful as a day-old kitten. So unless you're very experienced at this game, don't use gags, because it's extremely tempting to have a major-league panic once you realize you can't speak or see. A kidnapping scenario might sound like good, dangerous fun before you start, but games of control can have quite deep emotional effects and bring out all kinds of buried fears you never knew you had. You should tread carefully with it, and don't ever do anything you're not convinced is a great idea. So leave the gags to the professionals and make sure you're able to speak.

You may be of the belief that you'll look like a common hooker in a peep-hole bra and crotchless panties, but the only possible response to this is "so?" You will look unbelievably hot, and by presenting what you're offering in such an appealing and upfront fashion, you are basically telling him that you find him so attractive you want to show yourself off to the best advantage. It's much naughtier than straight nudity, and once in a while it doesn't hurt to get a little dirty—plus it means that if you're a bit lazy, you get to have sex without getting undressed.

harness

You can buy devices that give you the full dungeon effect in your own home without actually needing to construct a massive bunker under your house. Harnesses that fit over doors, for instance, which work like handcuffs but mean that you're hanging slightly off the floor—like a 17th-century prisoner—lend themselves to whipping and spanking games. I can't say it works for me, but hey, if you like the idea of being suspended by your wrists while your partner flogs you, go ahead, make your day. There are also harnesses that hold you in a position for easy access—your legs are parted and your arms are pinned down by the ankle and wrist straps that they feature—and submission is definitely the name of the game in one of these.

handing over control

You may find, if you take turns being dominant and submissive, that you both fall naturally into certain roles—which are often the opposite of your normal roles in the relationship. Powerful men, for instance, often like to be controlled sexually because it means they can hand over responsibility—and the same goes for women who wield power in normal life. It helps to decide on your scenario in advance—you don't have to go as far as writing a script, but having a vague idea of whether you're being Sub or Dom, and what the idea behind the scene is, makes it more convincing and enjoyable. Partly because it seems a bit silly to finish your evening meal, and then say, "So, should we go upstairs and whip each other senseless now?" Having a plot—however shaky and ill-thought-out—gives you more reason to be doing it, and helps you to shed your inhibitions more effectively. Even if it gets no further than "you've been a very naughty boy, now bend over." Useful scenarios include dungeon master/mistress and prisoner, virgin and evil tyrant, lord of darkness and slave … come on, it's not that difficult, is it?

If actual whipping seems a little harsh, there's no reason why you shouldn't give spanking a try. It's easier to control pain levels that way, as he—or you—can feel exactly how hard a hand is slapping bare ass, whereas with a cat o' nine tails whip you're not going to feel a thing except crazed with power. If it does get a little too painful, it's worth keeping some body lotion in the fridge, and rubbing it on the

---

TIP

Don't be shy about trimming your pubic hair—there's nothing wrong with it the way it is but it's pleasant to have a neat little triangle. And why stop there … you can trim it into a heart or a tiny Brazilian-waxed strip, which appeals to men reared on porn. Hell, snip it into a parallelogram for fun if you want to.

TIP

When you're dressing up, the idea is to keep at least some of your clothes on during sex—and as you will almost certainly be wearing stockings and garter belts, the vital thing to know is that you always put underwear on over the garters. I can't tell you the amount of trouble caused by couples wrestling with resistant elastic in a bid to expose enough flesh to actually have sex with each other—all because she put her panties on first. Discard the rest of the cheeky nurse's uniform if you must (must you?), but please, it's vital that you keep on your shoes and stockings … at least for a while.

---

red parts for a tingly sensation of relief, and, could it be … ah, yes! Must be arousing ….

After a certain period of time—could be ten minutes, could be hours—the game will almost always result in sex. But S&M-ers like to tease their partner to the point of orgasm, and then back away without letting them come—which is another form of mild torture. Eventually you'll be allowed your reward, but deferring the pleasure makes it even more enjoyable when it finally happens.

clubs

For the committed S&M-er, there's a whole social scene out there—and hey, who'd want to miss out on that? There are specialist stores devoted to the pastime, selling all kinds of whips, chains, and leather and rubber goods. And even more excitingly, there are social clubs devoted to aficionados of pain and pleasure.

But if you attend these members-only extravaganzas, you have to be prepared to see stuff that's hard to forget—couples whipping each other, naked and in public, group sex in giant spiders' webs, people hanging from manacles wearing rubber hoods … just like Sunday lunch at mom's, really. If you want to watch without joining in, it may be OK for a while—but unless your club welcomes voyeurs, you may be expected to get down and dirty yourselves. So be prepared.

watersports

Watersports are adventurous sex and then some. Well, some might say adventurous, others might just recoil in horror, murmuring, "How could you?" Most of us, we can admit, are probably of Group Two—because being peed on just doesn't do it for us. However, who are we to judge? And if you like the idea of being peed on, or peeing on someone else, you have every right to give it a whirl. The main attractions to devotees are the total lack of inhibition, the naughtiness of doing something forbidden, and the sensation of warmth and wetness it entails. Also, the urethra can become aroused if stimulated, so if he's playing with the hole, the urge to actually pee could be over-

---

TIP

Coming in your face is seen by some women as degrading—but if you're going to sit on his face, it seems only fair. They love it because accepting his semen all over you is tantamount to saying "I want the very essence of your manhood" (or as he might put it, "Yes! I want your hot come all over me, big boy!"). Either way, it's a sexy thing to do because it implies total acceptance. Kind of like if he lets you talk about shoes for a full hour when ESPN's announcing football scores. And it's only sperm—you can always wash it off.

---

whelming, so it's reassuring to know he won't run for the hills should you let it happen.

If you do, make sure you're doing it on a large plastic sheet. The carpet will never recover otherwise. Have a mop and bucket on hand so the smell isn't an issue (unless that turns you on ... oh dear), and drink plenty of water beforehand so your pee is a healthy straw color and relatively clean. Drinking pee is a really bad idea, whatever a bunch of alternative old hippies may think—so try to avoid it if possible. Apart from that, do whatever comes naturally, which tends to be one lying down and one standing up—or crouching—and doing the peeing. And hey, you kids enjoy yourselves, y'all hear?

threesomes & group sex

Here we come to the really risky bit of adventurous sex. It's all very well having fantasies about sleeping with another woman, or with two men—but if you decide to put it into practice, a warning siren should go off, and people in white hazmat suits should start running up

---

TIP

Mutual masturbation—which in this case means masturbating in front of each other—can be a big turn-on for both of you, as well as highly educational. It shows you exactly what each other likes. It takes a little courage to get going, but once you do, holding each other's gaze can be one of the sexiest things you'll ever do. If that feels too intimate, tape each other masturbating alone, and watch the videos together—believe me, no one will be embarrassed.

TIP

Watching other people have sex can be a real turn-on, but obviously, not that many people are up for it. You can, however, buy videos featuring actual, real people banging away at each other—renowned director Ben Dover also favors the unsophisticated porno technique, and makes films of ordinary-looking folk fucking in lighting that wouldn't disgrace the average convenience store. So if voyeurism is your bag (actually, a briefcase with a concealed camera in it is probably your bag)—check them out.

and down, spraying giant extinguishers and shouting, "Clear the building! Clear the building!" That's how dangerous it is. I'm not talking about nasty diseases—though that can be a concern. I'm talking about emotional nuclear meltdown. Jealousy is a powerful and vengeful god, and if you give it half a chance it can ruin your relationship—you know, the one you thought was totally secure? That one.

Watching your partner have sex or enjoy sexual intimacy with another person can be deeply traumatic—so even if you get drunk and think it'll be a real laugh, it might not be the next morning. If you're bisexual it could work—on the basis that you get all the fun and he hardly gets a peep. But what about the other woman? And what if he feels jealous? Because while "two women" is the fantasy of most men, "two women ignoring me" is not. The same goes for you—who wants to sit around watching her boyfriend getting off on someone else?

And if you decide it'd be a real laugh to take two men to bed, well, it might be as far as you're concerned. But unless your boyfriend

TIP

If you want the thrills of a threesome without risking your relationship, you can get a lot out of simply talking about it—describing what you'd do, and what the other man or woman would be doing to you both can be a turn-on, too. Don't either of you, however, discuss what his best friend or your sister would be doing—that can be a little too much information for most. This way, you can enjoy your fantasy together without the danger. Cowards!

is also bisexual it might simply spell complete jealousy and paranoia regarding sexual skills and penis size.

So you see why it's fraught with danger. But, having said all that, if a threesome (or even sixsome) is what you've always wanted and you're determined to try it, then there are ways of going about it that are less likely to end in total disaster. The "total disaster" way involves one of you falling in love with the third party. So to avoid that, it may be better if you don't choose someone you're already intimate with—his best friend, for instance. Bad idea. And you don't want to spend the rest of your life wondering if your own best friend is still secretly fantasizing about your partner's penis after one night of shared thrills. So to avoid all that (plus the ever-present danger of someone getting drunk and telling the packed local bar all about it), it's best to recruit a virtual stranger.

There used to be contact magazines for this sort of thing, and I always used to wonder how they did it once they'd made contact— "Brian and Sheila? Ted and Angela. Great. Now, have a few peanuts and a martini, then we can get our clothes off and fuck." I mean, really, how do you approach a complete stranger, or pair of strangers, and ask them if they'd like to have sex with you both? Luckily, the internet has been a godsend for swingers. There are endless chat rooms where you can meet like-minded people, and check out their photographs before you sign up for an intimate session with a three-hundred pound trucker from Ohio. Should things go well, you'll exchange e-mails. And then, once you're all best buddies—which may take a couple of days—you'll arrange to meet up. How things progress from there is up to you, but it will probably involve some sort of offer of a "massage." If your third party is very upfront, though, he or she may simply shake hands and get naked. Well, it's what you wanted, isn't it?

You'll need to agree on certain rules—whether that's "no kissing the other people" or "no intercourse with the others" or "everything's allowed, but we don't discuss it afterwards ...." Of course, I hardly need to tell you to use condoms. If you're advertising for sex on the net, chances are you're no virgin.

TIP

Take a leaf out of Sharon Stone's book—or at least Sharon Stone as she was in *Sliver* and *Basic Instinct*—and go out without panties, or else take them off while you're out and hand them to him as a little surprise present. Sharon did it, classily, under the table in the restaurant, which is always a good bet. If you chicken out, you can always run to the bathroom and then press them into his hot little hand. Knowing you're pantyless, even if he can't do anything about it, can lead to all sorts of filthy behavior later.

If you want to be more certain that you're getting a guy who isn't a total freak, however, you could try a male escort agency. That way, you'll have someone to complain to if he turns out to be a psychopath … just to look on the bright side.

If you're into real swinging, as in visiting swingers' clubs and mingling with other naked swappers, you can usually find details in contact magazines. But be very sure of your reasons for getting into the scene—and if you're having sex with other couples, the rules are, if either of you feels remotely uncomfortable, you stop right away, however much fun your partner's having—and you never make agreements to see one of your swappers behind your partner's back. Even if he has a bigger penis. Actually, especially if he's got a bigger penis.

exhibitionism

Exhibitionism is basically just sexual showing-off. It's sex where you're being watched, or you could be discovered—sex with a real risk. Both

---

TIP

If you decide to take a risk and go for sex outdoors, then choose your outfit with great care. In summer, it sounds dull, but covering yourself in insect repellent (then remembering not to lick it off) is also a useful precaution. Wear something long and floaty that you can drop to conceal yourself at a moment's notice, without underwear if possible. If you have to, a G-string is easier to push to one side than big panties—and no bra is a must. He has less options than you, but warm-ups with an easily-adjusted elastic waist are ultimately a lot more sensible than button-flies with a complex belt buckle when it comes to speedy dressing.

Masturbating in public is a fantasy that a lot of people share—but actually doing it risks upsetting a great many passersby and being arrested for indecent behavior. So a device that does the stimulating for you while no one knows is probably the answer. You can get super tiny (small enough to fit on a key chain) and relatively quiet (it runs on a watch battery) vibrators like the Itty Bitty. So, you're sitting on a boring car journey, you whip it out, pop it down your pants and off you go, with no one any the wiser. You could even try it in church—though I wouldn't recommend it. Duo-tone balls are a better bet there.

partners have to find the idea exciting for exhibitionist sex to work, though if one's a voyeur, the exhibitionist can masturbate while he or she watches—some will even have sex with another person while their partner watches, but that's not very common. If both of you are show-offs, though, it's a winner, since you'll both crave sex in supermarket parking lots.

Exhibitionism can be explored by taking pictures of each other—and sending them into the "Readers' Wives and Husbands" sections of porn mags. Then you can revel in how good you look next to the 45-year-old on the worn couch with the tits like beanbags—and imagine everyone else getting off on your picture, too. Once again, our old friend the internet plays a major part here—the world is the exhibitionist's oyster on the net. Webcams can record you undressing, masturbating or having sex and beam it out to a grateful nation for less than the price of a weekend in Cancún. And if you're a voyeur—well, there are enough exhibitionists out there to satisfy your every desire. The only concern is safety—which you can ensure by never giving your

TIP

If you really do feel like pushing the envelope exhibitionism-wise, you could do worse than try the popcorn jerk-off, which takes place in the theater. Wait till the lights go down—then he gets his dick out, makes a hole in the bottom of the box, sticks it through, and guides your hand right on in there. You don't have much room to maneuver, but that's really beside the point—it's the sheer naughtiness that's a turn-on. If you're nervous about being caught, though, go to an afternoon showing of a European art film rather than the 8:00 p.m. latest Tom Cruise flick. Just to be on the safe side.

personal details to anybody. And don't strip for the Webcam if the window behind you is right opposite the Empire State Building or anything recognizable—people can figure locations out surprisingly easily.

When it comes to having sex in public, swingers' clubs are the obvious port of call for the serious exhibitionist—no one's going to arrest you when half the guests are doing the same thing. If you get your jollies from giving him blow jobs in the middle of a mall, however, you need to be a little more careful. It's entirely likely you'll be arrested. Consider (slightly) safer options such as sitting on his lap at a nightclub wearing no undies and having sex while clubbers dance around you. Just don't get carried away and let anything slip ....

fetishism

A real fetish means you can't get aroused at all without your fetish object. It's usually men who develop fetishes and fixate their sexual feelings on a particular body part or object. Typical fetishes are shoes, feet, rubber, breasts—but they can go as far as car exhaust pipes, or even mud…. For the purposes of adventurous sex, however, you're probably just playing around with the idea of a fetish—it's not that you can't manage without, it's just that adding something else arousing to the sexual mix provides a lovely *frisson* once in a while. Say, for instance, high-heeled shoes with ankle straps. They elongate your legs, have a little hint of S&M about them, and most men find them hopelessly sexy. Or you could go for a transvestism fetish, and dress up as a man, while he dabs on make-up and puts on a dress. It may be a screamingly hilarious idea at first, but if he's a bit pretty it can bring out whole other aspects of your personalities—whether dominant, submissive, feminine, masculine, you can really play around with roles in your sexual relationship.

Rubber, too, can be a highly sexy possibility—the true fetish often begins with the rubbery pants that children wear to protect their clothes from "accidents"—sometimes men come to associate it with

---

TIP

If you are making a porno, certain positions lend themselves to looking sexy on film—and guess what, it's not missionary. You leaning up against a wall, face-first, with your back arched so your ass sticks out looks great on film—and so does doggy style because, to be blunt, it makes every woman's ass look fantastic. Typical porn poses show you off to best advantage, and allow the camera to pick up his penis going in and out— normal TV puts 10 pounds on, so maybe porn TV puts 10 inches on. There's always hope.

Keep the script short and to the point. Remember, the whole reason for making your porn film is to turn yourselves on watching it later. A lot of hot air—"My radiator's broken, can you fix it?" "Well, I don't know, I might need a wrench for that." "Do you have one in the van?" "I dunno, I'll go and look"—is not a sexy script. "God, I want to have you now" is more effective when it comes to scripting.

feelings of comfort and naughtiness. But even if the nearest you've ever got to rubber is a pencil eraser and your math homework, the sensation of it on your skin can be arousing. It's warm yet tight, and completely smooth. Rubber outfits can be very sexy—though if you're both rolling around in them, you'll be squeaking like a cageful of mice.

Fetishism can include black stockings, leather boxers (for him), full nurses' outfits, or even bandages. The good news is, when you both like it, you're both doing it in privacy, and so long as you're not nailing his penis to a plank of wood, with adventurous sex it really is a case of whatever (legally) turns you on ....

7 advanced sex

Having advanced sex isn't actually that different from having un-advanced sex—it just means you'll do it more smoothly, your orgasms will be enhanced, and the whole thing will resemble the difference between drunkenly trying to dance the macarena by copying the person in front of you, and actually learning how to do it and under-standing when you should jump in the air and put your hands on your shoulders. Ideally, though, the kind of sex you'll be having will provide you with slightly more fun than the macarena—unless, that is, you're a really, really good dancer.

advanced kissing

I know we said right at the start that kissing is easy. It is, you really don't need to practice. But advanced kissing is slightly more complex. There are many different types of kisses—from "Hi Gran," to the kind of nose-rub that means "Brother Inuit, there is drifting snow on the tundra and the seals are dying," to "Oh my god, my house, family and possessions are all going up in flames, but this feels so good I just can't bring myself to care." So to improve your own smooching reper-toire, focus on the subtleties of kissing.

Some believe there's a nerve that links the upper lip to the geni-tals—and who are you to prove them wrong? By nibbling on the lip, you can send messages of lust right through his body—so do it for a while, won't you?

You can also indulge in butterfly kisses—typically, fluttering your eyelashes on his skin—but it can also mean tiny, featherlike kisses all over his face, finally concentrating on the corners of his mouth, and along his lips.

Then there's the Snake kiss—where you flick the tip of your tongue in and out between his lips and make brief contact with the tip of his tongue before pulling out again.

And the Soul kiss, where your tongues entwine and you breathe into each other's mouths. Or even the kiss that is more of a suck—you suck on his lower lip, he sucks on your upper lip, and according to some *Kama Sutra*–toting sources, you can even have an orgasm this way. It may take a while, though.

advanced foreplay

understanding each other's bodies

For good sex, it's essential that you understand how each other's bodies respond. When he touches your neck, you may experience an entirely different sensation from the one he feels when you touch his. And while you may love to have your nipples played with, for him it may just feel weird and slightly annoying. So it's worth devoting quite some time to practicing different touches and caresses on different parts of each other. Techniques include stroking, biting, sucking, licking, pinching and rubbing. Sex expert Anne Hooper calls this process "body mapping." She suggests that couples take turns blindfolding each other, and use a scale of numbers to judge arousal—if they feel nothing, it's -3, if it's practically orgasmic, it's a +3—a very handy way for your partner to know what's worth bothering with and what

If his penis is on the small side, then a handy tip is to wait until it's really big before you let him enter you—and the best way to maximize penis potential is by sucking it, hard. Once you really don't believe it can get any bigger without a vacuum pump, roll a ribbed condom over it—this will create the friction that may be lacking from a really small one. And if you also adopt one of the "deep entry" positions—which you'll know if you've been paying attention—you'll barely know the difference between him and an average-sized guy. Obviously, don't mention that.

isn't. Focus on one small area at a time, and concentrate fully on the sensations you're feeling.

stroking

Stroking is perfect for a general relaxation session. He should stroke you by alternating small, brushing motions and big, sweeping motions all over. Your back, butt, thighs—both inner and outer—and arms will probably respond well to stroking. When it's his turn, focus on the sides of his torso—a highly neglected area—inner thighs and his butt. Many men are less sensitive in their limbs than women are, so don't waste endless time trailing your fingers up and down his calves, it's probably not worth your while.

biting

If you use it carefully, biting can be intensely erotic. Make sure you take your cue from your partner when it comes to how hard to clamp your teeth together, though—an arousing nip is not the same thing as a blood-drawing chew. Good places for biting on you are your neck just below your ears and at the back—gently—your earlobes, butt cheeks, inner thighs, and your sides. Biting breasts is rarely a good plan, unless he does it as if he were holding a little baby fairy between his teeth. And even then, go easy. On him, earlobes, inner thighs, neck, butt, sides—all can benefit from light biting.

sucking

The main focus of attention here is almost certainly going to be breasts. He should suck gently, though, not as if he's trying to unclog a sink. And he can also try it on your thighs, fingers (very erotic), earlobes and—if he's inclined to—toes. You should suck his—well, obviously his penis, but it's hardly news that that feels good, is it?—fingers (because it reminds him of having his penis sucked), earlobes, balls and—if you're up to it—toes.

licking

Licking is good news as far as your neck, ears, collarbone, breasts, butt, back and thighs are concerned. In fact, there are few places that don't benefit from a nice little lick. He should run his tongue down your spine, flicker it into the crevice at the top of your buttocks, and circle the tip lovingly on your inner thighs. You, meanwhile, should focus your licking efforts on his neck, ears, nipples, hips, butt, balls and inner thighs. That's a lot of tongue work ….

pinching

Pinching can be oddly arousing—if it's done lightly and in the right places. It's good for your butt, nipples and inner thighs—on him, the same is probably true. Pinching anywhere else just looks like cruelty—and don't even think about trying it with his penis.

rubbing

Some people are so sensitive that if you rub them too hard in one spot they'll develop a sore spot—which is really not what you want at all. But a little gentle rubbing can work wonders on necks, inner elbows, back of knees, spines—and here is where feet come into their own because while you may not want to bite, nibble or suck them, almost everyone loves having their feet rubbed.

By understanding exactly what works when it comes to touching each other, you'll ensure that you don't waste hours poking and prodding in the completely wrong places, wondering why you aren't getting the response you hoped for. What's more, your foreplay will be streamlined so perfectly that your partner may well be trembling on the verge of an orgasm before you even reach their genitals. Which is a good thing.

advanced orgasm

Okay, sit up and pay attention. An advanced orgasm is not as difficult as it sounds. But it turns out there are different types. According to Lou Paget, men can experience an orgasm in up to seven different ways, and women in up to ten different ways. Now, don't feel insecure about this. It's merely to give you an inkling of the possibilities; nobody's suggesting you should be having ten different kinds of orgasm or else you're not enjoying yourself—fun's fun, and if it feels good, just one kind's fine by most of us. But just so you know, the ways men can experience orgasm are, apparently, via intercourse, manual, oral, prostate, fantasy/dreams, touching or sucking breasts,

The two-handed hand job is a winner because it ensures that your clit feels great, without putting any excess pressure on it—this one works very well if you've had a lot of stimulation lately (I know, you should be so lucky) and your clitoris can't take any direct action. He just needs to place one hand over the other, then put both of them over your pubic mound and rub slowly. The spreading of pressure across a wider area means that you'll get new, thrilling sensations but you won't orgasm for a while, which may suit you just fine.

and sex toys. Doesn't sound that complicated now, does it? Although most men past the age of 14 might have trouble coming from just breast contact alone. As for women, they can orgasm via clitoral, vaginal and cervical (no, I don't know what the big difference is there, either) stimulation, G-spot, urethra, breast contact, mouth contact, anal, blended/fusion, zone and fantasy.

Alright, now we really are in the realms of sci-fi. It's just about acceptable that certain very specific individual women may possibly be able to come through merely being kissed. We suspect, however, that these women are lonely nuns, suddenly surprised by manly motorcyclists who have roared into the convent grounds and crushed the startled sisters against their hard, leather-clad chests ... hang on, I'm beginning to understand ... fair enough. But Blended and Fusion? Zone? Are these orgasms or diets, for goodness sake?

In truth, it's relatively simple. Ish. A Blended or Fusion orgasm means that more than one area of the body is being stimulated. I bet you never knew that his playing with your nipple and your clitoris simultaneously had a special grown-up name, did you? Well, now you do. A Zone orgasm, meanwhile, just means you've orgasmed from having an area of the body stimulated that wouldn't normally lead to an orgasm. So if he's rubbing your nose and suddenly you're overcome with waves of pulsating sensation, you'll know you've had a Zone orgasm. Or, possibly, you've sneezed.

his and hers

It should be becoming clear by now that men and women have markedly different experiences of orgasm. Which is why a simultaneous orgasm is so rare. Forget all the films you've ever seen where they're at it like ferrets in a bag, then suddenly they both go all eye-rolling and start shouting "uh! Yes! Oh god!" and collapse in a heap at the same time. She's so faking it. Well, so is he, he's acting, but if they were real people she would be, too. A simultaneous orgasm hardly ever happens through penetration, though it can occasionally occur through mutual masturbation as long as you speed it up and then slow it down to match your partner's rate of arousal. Which makes sex sound about as exciting as test-driving a Geo Prism, but still. And if he is still blathering on about why you aren't having multiple, award-winning orgasms during sex, you may wish to point out that 28% of women can't come at all during sex, with or without clitoral stimulation. Though I couldn't begin to imagine how they found that out—"Excuse me, ma'am, we're conducting a survey ...."

Anyhow, the joy of simultaneous orgasm is a myth. Because even if you do manage to achieve one, you're both so busy galloping along your own little racetracks to the finishing line you don't pay any attention to each other—and surely at least part of the point of sex is to enjoy your partner's responses?

The best way to do it, if possible, is for you to come first, and then let him come. Otherwise, he'll come, then go all comatose and sleepy because he's been flooded with dopamine, and you'll be left to finish the job yourself, whether you like it or not. Oh, he'll make some half-hearted hand-flapping attempt, but if you want to be sure of decent orgasms all around, try to get yours in first.

advanced anatomy

It's not that you need a degree in advanced human biology to enjoy sex or anything—but it's nice to be able to pinpoint the important bits of your inner workings, should the need arise. So with that in mind, here's a quick refresher course on where to find all those spots ... let's call it the Dalmatian Course.

g-spot

You'll find this around 2 inches up on the front inner wall of the vagina. It's an area of soft, ridgy or spongy tissue, the size of a nickel, but it swells to ... ooh, at least a quarter ... when correctly stimulated. If you're looking for it (and hey, aren't we all, honey?) you need to squat on all fours right after stimulation, so it's engorged and easier to locate—then get your fingers right up there and wiggle them around. Or he can.

a-spot

It's farther up than the G-spot, another spongy little spot, on the front inner wall again. To find it—you may need a dildo or extra-long pianist's fingers for this—use a light pressing motion on the front wall, and push down with your abdominal muscles to heighten the

TIP

When searching for the G-spot, it helps if you go to the bathroom first. Otherwise, all that prodding about near the bladder can prove highly distracting since it puts pressure on the sphincter muscles, and suddenly you'll need the toilet just as things are getting good. Some women like the sensation of a full bladder and find it increases their chances of orgasm—but if you're not one of them, make sure you go before you go, as your gran used to say. Though she probably didn't mean it like that.

sensations. Leaning backward may help—but if you can't find it, you're in good company.

c-spot

This is the spot right at the neck of your cervix—and you need to go very carefully here, because banging around there can hurt. After all, pap smears aren't the biggest laugh going, are they? But if you get it right, you can experience deep and giddy sensations from the C-spot. Getting it right, however, takes effort. Try hooking your ankles over his shoulders and raising your butt so you're tipped backward— that's about as deep as penetration gets, and you stand a fair chance of bumping it—but tell him to go gently. Easier is an extra-long vibrator with a rounded tip, which may well stimulate the spot in question through gentle buzzing.

u-spot

It's surrounded on three sides by the clitoris and its environs, so stimulation here is sure to result in some kind of excitement, even if it does make you want to pee. He can locate this one for you in a most pleasant fashion by placing his lower lips over his teeth during oral sex and applying light pressure on the spot in question. And it will respond remarkably well to a soft, gentle tongue stroke.

female ejaculation

We all know about male ejaculation. It's called semen, it contains sperm, it looks like ectoplasm, and it goes everywhere when you give hand jobs. Simple. Female ejaculation, however, is a whole different ballgame. There is controversy as to whether it actually exists—some think it's pee, but there is definitely a colorless fluid that can be ejaculated from the vagina at the point of orgasm. It may simply be lubrication that's collected in a pool, and a muscle spasm shoots it out at once ... who knows, it may be pixies' special lemonade, whatever, but if you want to try it, you need to be aroused to the point of orgasm, then as you feel the first contraction, bear down hard with your abdominal muscles, as though you're trying to shoot peas off your stomach. It may or may not happen—but there's no harm in trying.

TIP

When giving him a blow job, twist your tongue around the tip every time you come up the shaft. You don't need to be too rhythmic—just alternate between clockwise and counterclockwise, or swirl it around as if you're licking a waffle cone packed with delicious ice cream. The contrast between your sucking action and the little extra swirling sensation on the most sensitive area should make him forget why penises were invented in the first place—he'll believe it was simply for this.

If you want to swallow when you give him a blow job, certain foods make his semen taste much better—and the best thing he can drink to improve the flavor is pineapple juice. Maybe give him some coconut milk, too, then you'll get the whole pina colada thing going on … but the enzymes in pineapple juice have a sweetening effect on his secretions, so force it down him. Foods he should avoid include tobacco, caffeine and asparagus. You can also try going down on him with a swig of mild mouthwash—it's exciting for him, and masks the taste of any asparagus-based semen for you.

advanced oral sex

Oral sex? Come on, surely you know it all by now! But wait, there's still a little information that may be to your advantage ….

69

69 position … been there, done that? You sure? OK, but did you enjoy it? That's the trouble with 69, it really is way too much like rubbing your tummy and patting your head. It's far too complicated to get comfortable enough to enjoy a real, relaxed orgasm—you're too busy trying to avoid getting a cramp in your neck, or your jaw seizing up, and he's struggling to breathe. But that's the classic 69 position, where you lie with your bodies alongside each other, you've got your head stuffed between his legs, he's got his stuffed between yours, and that's not accounting for the fact that both your bodies are jack-knifed uncomfortably due to the height difference between you.

> **TIP**
>
> Men can actually strengthen their tongues in the same way they can practice to strengthen their PC muscles. A particularly useful exercise to get his tongue used to moving in a different way from its usual pattern of tasting chips and beer and talking is for him to lick out a container of yogurt. The necessity of extracting every last drop will mean he has to extend his tongue like a python and rotate it gently—which is excellent practice when he comes to do the same for your own, um, yogurt cup ….

This is not the best way to get the most out of it. What you should be doing is this: You lie on your back, and he crouches above you, facing your feet. That way you get to give him a blow job and play with his balls, which are miraculously accessible, and he gets to go down on you upside down, which is highly enjoyable, and means he can also reach a finger into your vagina.

You can do the position in reverse—you crouching over him— but that involves slightly more work for you, which is obviously less desirable.

blow job

For the ultimate blow job, it works best if you're crouching between his legs while he sits on the edge of the bed, or a chair. He can stand and lean against a wall, if he prefers. Being on your knees may be a little subservient but it gives you a lot more room to move. That way, too, he can look down and see exactly what your tongue is doing. With one hand, reach underneath to caress his balls, and form your mouth into a hard "o" for the best sensation you can offer. If your lips are too floppy you could be there for hours getting a numb jaw. The best way to bring matters to a swift conclusion is with strong, power-ful sucking action—it may be a little harsh on the cheeks but he'll appreciate it so much it's almost worth it. Move your head back and forth, and, in the meantime, flicker your tongue across the tip of his penis, and up and down, quickly and lightly. When he starts to make "about to come" noises, don't stop—this is not the time to pull away and say "are you about to come in my mouth?" Just keep on truckin' and—yes—let him come in your mouth, swallow, and even try and pretend you enjoyed it. Easy.

cunnilingus

The ultimate is simply getting it right, which is harder than it sounds. But to give you the best blow job you've ever had, he needs to bear a few things in mind. Lying right between your legs is out—but lying with his head at right angles, so it's pillowed on your thigh and his fingers can reach in to spread your labia, is definitely in. To make it easier for him, you can raise your other leg to give him more access. He should begin with the Kivin method (see Chapter 3 for details)

TIP

If he's going down on you, it's vital he shaves first—unless he has enough stubble growth to make it soft. If he does, pressing his chin lightly against your vagina will create a series of prickles that feels fantastic as he moves his face. Which he should do—far too many men seem to think they have to assume one head position and use their tongue to do all the work, whereas actually moving his head around allows him much greater access to all your nooks and crannies. Hence the need not to have ago-nizingly painful stubble.

before moving on to stimulate the U-spot with soft gentle licks. Circling movements are required, and he shouldn't take his tongue away. At the same time, he can insert a finger in your vagina to press on the G-spot, and press another against your anus. He can, if he has the coordination of a Russian ice dancer, reach his other hand up and play with your breasts and nipples. As long as he remembers the catchwords "light" and "gentle" it can only be a matter of minutes before a shattering orgasm overtakes you.

"hovering butterfly"

Sitting on his face—or, by its more sensitive name, "hovering butterfly"—is more a matter of suspending yourself above his face. If you actually sat on it, he'd suffocate, which may be an admirable way to go, but is perhaps a little unnecessarily dramatic. The best way to do it is by holding onto something behind his head—like the headboard—otherwise your thigh muscles will go into spasm halfway through. If there's nothing to hold onto, lean forward, and put your hands on the wall. The beauty of this position is that he has full access both visually and physically—he can part your labia with his fingers and see exactly what he's doing and where with his tongue. He can also reach your breasts and butt—so if you can overcome your inhibitions, face-sitting is a great way to enjoy advanced oral sex. Note, however, that him sitting on your face really doesn't work—unless you're doing the whole anal thing.

how to delay male orgasm

Since at least half this book is dedicated to the pursuit of orgasm, it seems a little strange to be attempting to put it off. But some men—

though not many women—do suffer from the curse of premature ejaculation, which means that nobody's having quite as much fun as they could. There are, however, ways of avoiding this—chief among them being the stop-start technique.

He enters you and thrusts to the point just before orgasm is inevitable. Then he pulls out, waits for the feelings to subside for a few seconds—he can continue to touch you while he waits, though—and then re-enters you, carries on again till he feels an orgasm approaching like a runaway train, then pulls out again …. This can continue until you're both satisfied, at which point he's finally allowed to come.

Another method, if you can't be bothered with all the stopping and starting, or if he doesn't have a problem with it but you just want to go on longer, is the Squeeze technique. Just before he comes, make a ring around the base of his penis with your thumb and forefinger and squeeze lightly. This should stop the semen that thinks it's on its way to victory, and buy you a little more time. But really, don't squeeze too hard. That's just mean.

TIP

One simply lovely tip to hold back male orgasm is for him to imagine he's taking a crap and activate the same muscles (but not so much that he really … oh god, oh god, stop there). This has the interesting effect of preventing orgasm, in much the same way as images of nuns, or grannies in big undies, are alleged to. For you, however, if you want to encourage an orgasm, the best thing you can do with your muscles is to clench your lower stomach hard, as your excitement begins to peak. This can intensify and prolong your orgasm—if you just forget the fact that he's thinking about crap.

advanced sex toys

As was seen in Chapter 5, the world of sex toys has many places to explore—and new ones are constantly being designed. Ultimately, they're all there to ensure your orgasm—but the routes they offer to get you there are increasingly fascinating. Toys specially designed for anal sex, which feature a flange to stop them from lodging in your rectum, are available—not to mention the Hot Rod, with a slim (as small as seven-eighths of an inch in diameter), angled shaft and a rounded shaft that you can either wear in a harness or use manually … I'd love to have been at the marketing meeting for these things. You can also get a vibrating "tail spin," a dildo that offers a tail that spins gently inside your anus. It sounds a little too much like some kind of weird butt-toothbrush to be truly sensual, but it may be worth a try.

For vaginal/clitoral excitement, however, you may want to invest in a vibrating love cushion, which does exactly what it says—you switch it on, sit on it, and before you know it, you're having wild orgasms with no hands involved. It feels kind of like when the bus stops and the engine's still on, only better. And without the school kids throwing backpacks around.

The Tongue Joy, meanwhile, is a vibrating bullet-shaped attachment that fixes to your tongue with a little strap and allows anywhere you lick to also be vibrated. It may feel weird for the user, but it feels damn hot for the one experiencing it. Just don't swallow it in your excitement.

There are also specially designed cock rings, with clit stimulators attached. Try the Bump-N-Grind, which has a holding dock for an Itty

Bitty. Hell, you can even get the Foxy Vibe butt plug, a cute little device shaped like a fox perched on a log. Insert a vibrator into its hollow notch and the ears vibrate. Feels great and so adorable looking!

advanced thrusting

Thrusting isn't that difficult—all he has to do is plunge in and out, aided by your hip movements, in a bid to create friction. Anyone can, and does, do it. Advanced thrusting, however, relies on maintaining a certain level of control. He needs to build up his PC muscle by hanging a washcloth on his penis and raising and lowering it—look, good sex takes work, you know.

But by learning to control his speed and power of thrust, he can improve the sexual experience for both of you. Try it with several short thrusts, followed by one sudden, deep thrust—the more unexpected, the better it is for you, but don't try it in a deep-penetration position; it's best in missionary.

You can also train your PC muscles to the extent that you can have sex without moving, once he's inside you. You sitting on top is the best position by far for this. He inserts his penis inside you and you squeeze it with your vagina in a series of short contractions. The stronger the muscles, the better it will feel for him—if they're gladiator-strength, you can make him come this way, but it takes a lot of practice. He'll thank you for it, though.

You can also enjoy slower, more erotic sex by rotating your hips together, rather than thrusting—this has the added effect of grinding on your clitoris and stimulating the full area of your vaginal wall.

advanced roleplay

With fantasy, as stated in Chapter 4, the only thing to bear in mind is whether your partner actually wants to know or not. If not, you're somewhat hampered when it comes to acting it out. If so, however, there's little to stop you, except the fear that it won't be as good in real life. The truth is, you're right, it might not be. But one fantasy nearly always works as a roleplay—the Strangers in the Night fantasy. Having sex with a stranger is one of the top fantasies enjoyed by both men and women. Although he or she may be faceless—and fantasy lovers often are—it's the knowledge that you won't be judged, nobody will know, and that you can be completely uninhibited that gives the imaginary encounter its excitement, unhampered by relationship issues, insecurities and real life. It's a simple transaction of desire and being desired in its most basic form. Now, if you were to enact this in real life, your partner would, understandably, be thoroughly annoyed, and may well leave you. As a shared fantasy, however, it's perfectly possible to act it out, highly convincingly.

You need to arrange—via text message, if possible, to make it detached—to both be in a hotel bar at a certain time. You must arrive separately—it's no use setting out together. He arrives first, books a room, and settles down in the bar in the manner of a jaded business traveler. You get all dressed up, shave your legs, wax your pubic hair (unless that gives you a nasty rash) and generally prepare to go on the prowl. Then, you turn up in the bar and take a separate table. After a while, he sends a drink over to your table. You smile in acknowledge-ment … and after a while, you invite him over. You talk about any-thing but your personal lives—and you don't ever crack a smile of complicity, or let on that this is a game—you'll ruin it. Saying "just a minute, did you pick up the dry-cleaning?" will be the end of everything.

After a while, you start flirting … big-time. Others in the bar will watch as you fondle his knee and he strokes your arm. And they will watch open-mouthed as you head for the elevator together, then proceed to the room he's booked and have mind-blowing sex. Afterwards, you may want to end the game. Or you may want to carry on, leave, return to him, and greet him the next day without ever mentioning your night of illicit passion in the arms of a stranger.

advanced behavior

Sexual behavior that's not advanced is no longer part of your repertoire, of course. But there's just a couple more things that need mentioning. Like, initiating sex. Far too many couples rely on the man to do all the initiation—then they wonder why they fall into a pattern where he's pestering, and she's whining and moaning about being tired. If you make a conscious effort, however, to initiate it yourself—and you'd be depressed to learn how few long-term couples actually bother to kiss more than once every few weeks—you'll be amazed at how much it perks up your sex life. He'll feel wanted, you'll feel sensual and uninhibited, and those feelings will miraculously translate into your sex life.

8 spiritual sex

Spiritual sex is the kind you don't have with a one-night stand. While it can be passionate, its whole point is about forging a deeper connection between you. Staring into each other's eyes is par for the course, but you'll also be expected to breathe into each other's mouths, and generally unite in a bubble of one-ness on the path to orgasm. The reward for all this intimacy and patience is, of course, the greatest orgasm known to man—the full body orgasm, or FBO, as those in the know like to call it.

Along the way, though, you should grow in your spiritual understanding of each other—and ideally, learn how not to feel silly while pulling a penis to unleash the chi energy. Actually, that might be something you have to come to terms with yourself.

Some of the moves are a direct descendant from yoga—and others are connected to the Eastern philosophies and their belief in chi energy points, or chakras. Basically, this is not the sexual technique you'll want for a quickie.

connecting with your sexual energy

Non-tantric sex has a beginning, middle and end—it's a very linear process, which goes from arousal to plateau to orgasm, and it can take less than 15 minutes. In fact, as we all know, occasionally it can take less than 5. And given that a lot of women need a good 20 minutes (or even a very average 20 minutes) to reach full arousal, that can't be good.

Tantric sex, by contrast, is approached as circular activity—there's no designated final credits where "The End" rolls in loopy writing over a scene with the two of you sharing a cigarette. The "being in the moment of union" is what it's all about—experiencing every sensation fully, without leaping ahead to the end as fast as possible. The good part is that it's not all just look-into-my eyes stuff—it also regularly features several orgasms in a single session. No wonder Sting always looks so relaxed.

For spiritual sex you need to build up your sexual energies by slowing the process right down. In your case, you can begin to prepare by slowly massaging your breasts—start at the edges and work inward in small, slow circles. This apparently keeps your mind focused on

---

TIP

A Taoist exercise called the Golden Circle can help you to direct sexual energy from the pelvic area through the rest of the body. Sit with your eyes closed and relax your tongue so it sits just behind your teeth, then focus your attention on your pelvic girdle—it's the bones of your hips, pubic area and lower back, and it's bowl-shaped. Visualize it filled with warm golden honey, then imagine it flowing in a tube from your spine to the top of your head. When it reaches the top, hold your breath for five seconds, then breathe out as it flows back down. Hold it for a minute as it reaches the bowl again. Don't strain—just stop for a moment if it's not happening for you. The idea is to move chi through your body, and your imagination can help its flow.

---

the sex organs—but it also encourages the flow of blood to your breasts and makes them increase in size. It's called a chi massage, and the male version requires him to rub his perineum and massage his testicles with two fingers, using a light, gentle stroke, for several minutes.

He should then grasp the end of his penis—not an instruction that many men resent—while breathing out, and bend over, pushing his tongue out and pulling on his penis. Yes, it does look hilariously stupid. But if it builds up sexual energy, then who are you to argue with the ancient Taoists? The exercises aren't done with the aim of viewing intercourse as the goal—it's merely a staging post along the way to Nirvana, alright?

And there are certain things you need to do before you even think about having sex that will ensure that when you do it's a thing of beauty and a joy forever.

The first stage is to find out what turns your partner on—without expecting that the discussion will turn into sex. You're expected

---

TIP

Your skin is your biggest erogenous zone, and breast skin is particularly thin and therefore sensitive—so he shouldn't ignore its potential. Going straight for the nipples means missing out on a whole world of stimulation, when he should be swirling his fingertips across the skin of your breasts and tracing them along the underside to awaken a whole bunch of nerves you never even knew were there. Stroking, however, is not the same thing as squashing—so make sure he doesn't start treating them like Play-Doh.

Women prefer wildly differing strengths of nipple suction, so to make sure that he isn't treating them like he's trying to get an extra-thick milkshake through a cocktail straw, just suck on his tongue to show him what you'd like him to do. You could suck on his nipples, but they're less sensitive than yours, whereas his tongue is highly sensitive—unless he's a heavy smoker who exists on loads of chili peppers … in which case you probably don't want to be going anywhere near his mouth.

to make your relationship a priority—even if you have kids, or highly demanding careers, and can't spare the time that would have been available to a courtesan of an ancient emperor. You can still set aside at least an hour or two a week to devote to yourselves, without the TV or the children blaring in the background. You will also be expected to make the atmosphere reasonably pleasant—so rendezvousing in a bedroom overflowing with laundry and old newspapers will do bad things, feng shui wise. You may not be able to turn it into the required "sacred space" with five minutes and only a trash bag at your disposal, but you can certainly light some candles and stick a few flowers in a vase. Scented candles are ideal since the relaxing or sensual ones will put you in the mood much faster than the smell of next door's fried chicken. At the very least, switch a lamp on instead of that glaring overhead 60-watt thing, and play some suitable music.

Pay attention to what you wear, too—worn-out jogging shorts aren't perhaps the most sensual of outfits for either of you. Or have baths or showers first—a good plan anyway—and turn up in the manner of Marilyn Monroe, wearing nothing but Chanel No. 5. He will, of course, be wearing aftershave. Accessorize yourself with jewelry, long, seductive earrings or necklaces.

intimacy

Ritual is used in tantra to develop intimacy—not your normal ritual, however, of "where's the remote?," "you're sitting on it," "do you want a cup of coffee?"—but a far more seductive one. At least, we can only hope so.

Food is a good basis for ritual—and finger food is even better because you can feed each other. Obviously, we're not talking about scrambled eggs or sausages, but seductive food like fruit, asparagus (though it does make his come taste terrible) and chocolates. Wine is also a good bet at this point, to overcome any lingering inhibitions, plus it's been used in rituals of one sort or another since time immemorial. Or your ritual could be as simple as bathing together in scented water.

As long as you're focusing on each other positively, whether that takes the form of a game of cards or a prolonged poetry-reading session, you're on the right track.

If you're really into the whole idea of tantric sex, you'll be doing this for some weeks before you consider moving onto sex—it's all about building up the anticipation, though you may feel that's pushing things a bit far. Hey, I'm only telling you what some people do ....

breathing control

Do you ever think about breathing? It's unlikely, it being simply a matter of processing enough air in and out to stay alive. But in tantric sex breathing matters, trust me. Shared breathing is a powerful way to bring you closer and help you focus on each other. Sit facing each other cross-legged. Put your hands on your knees, palms up, and look into your partner's eyes, taking slow, deep breaths. You may feel like a complete dork, but it's worth doing, honest.

Breathe at the same rate, in through your nose and out through your mouth (you can chant "in with anger, out with love" at the same time if you want to, but probably not). Ideally, you'll be able to maintain this breathing, coupled with eye contact, for a good 10 minutes or so. Then and only then are you allowed to touch each other. It's alleged that some couples achieve orgasm through "soul gazing" alone. I'm sure they have, and I'd love to meet them.

erotic touch

You are now allowed to touch—hurrah! But it's back to Anne Hooper's body mapping, not wild sex—you're just touching each other gently and talking about what feels good. Tell each other where you want to be stroked or caressed, whether you'd prefer it to be with fingers or tongue, and be appreciative when each other gets it right.

According to tantric teaching, the longer you build up sexual energy, the longer men can avoid orgasming. Start your actual lovemaking session by kissing each other all over—it's important that you don't start breathing heavily, like a marathon runner, as soon as the excitement kicks in. Panting hurries you toward orgasm, but deep, slow, measured breaths will hold it off. If you now start breathing alternately—he breathes out as you breathe in—you'll be more connected.

If you are breathing into each other's mouths though, be careful—you don't want to build up so much carbon dioxide you'll feel faint and dizzy. At least not for any reason other than lust.

positions

In tantra, different positions are used to increase pleasure as well as balancing chi energy. So men are expected to take female "subservient" roles as well as the more traditional dominant ones, which frees them to engage on a more emotional level, while you can be more direct and demanding than is traditionally expected. Of course, nowadays, that's not so unusual, but come on—at the time it was wild. So you might adopt the traditional missionary, but with the positions reversed, so you're leaning over him, or he might be the inner "spoon" that fits to your body while you caress his penis.

All that Flaying of the Goat *Kama Sutra* stuff is not strictly necessary—I mean, you can if you want, but tantra isn't about bending your legs behind your ears, it's about making a connection.

multiple for men

Orgasm and ejaculation are separate in tantra world and we already know that he can come without actually ejaculating. But the exciting bit is, rather than just showing off and allowing his sperm to end up lying around in his bladder instead of on the sheet, by doing this he can experience a series of mini-orgasms within a controlled climax. According to tantra, he is simply surfing the energy wave, without drowning in it. To do this, he can put various tricks—I mean, modes of tantric enlightenment—into practice. He can clench the PC muscles, as explained in Chapter 3, in a series of short bursts. He can also consciously relax. As soon as he feels his orgasm overtaking him he should take a deep breath and pause in his thrusting—similar to the stop-start technique. Don't let his erection collapse altogether, though.

TIP

If his penis is bigger than your vaginal opening it may cause problems. Don't be alarmed—your vagina can stretch—but it's vital that you allow lots of time for foreplay. One useful way to handle it, though, is for you to come before he tries to penetrate you—a relaxed vagina makes an enormous difference as to how easy it is to get inside. Ensuring you're fully wet and relaxed will be a lot less painful when he tries. He should go slowly, though, and the best position is woman on top, so you can control the speed and depth of the thrusting.

If he tightens his PC muscles every time his arousal peaks, it should hold off orgasm for quite some time. In fact, you could still be there next Tuesday wondering when he'll finally get around to it. To have his flow of mini-orgasms, he needs to finally clench his PCs and take a deep breath at the same time—it's hard to pick the exact moment, though, so don't be surprised if it all goes pear- (or ectoplasm-) shaped a few times first. When he gets it, though, he'll be ecstatic … and you'll be … well, presumably concentrating on your own orgasm.

your tantric orgasm

Obviously, clitoral stimulation is expected—no, demanded. But the old G-spot rears its spongy head again here because in tantra it's known as the Sacred Spot. So yes, once again you'll be unfolding the map and hoping for the best—only this time, it's spiritual. A good grasp of tantra should mean that you can direct energy through the body's chakras, which builds up sensations of heightened pleasure.

ways of touching

Tantric touching is the key to all pleasure (oh, apart from breathing) and it's important that you change the style of your touching every minute or so—except during oral sex, that is, in which case the rule is, if it ain't broke, don't fix it. Alternating touch, however, builds up sexual energy. It's useful to look for areas of each other's bodies that feel cool, then caress them till they warm up—that way you release even more energy. In fact, you're releasing so much by now you could probably bottle it and sell it as Tantric Viagra.

where to begin

Start your touching with each other's faces, where the nose meridian is connected to the root chakra. Extend your stroking downward, through each other's necks, arms, breasts/torso, stomach, genitals, and then go back, completing the body-circle of touching—even if he's begging you to stick with the genitals. By doing this you're creating an energy circuit. See, it's just like physics.

For you, he should gently suck and lick your upper lip so his lower lip rubs against the connecting tissue between your gums and upper lips—this apparently has a direct line to the clitoris. You may not orgasm from this alone, but there's no harm trying, is there?

For him, stimulate the area where his shoulders join his neck. This part responds very well to biting and nibbling, and even sucking. You need to move up the back of the neck to the base of the skull—doing this releases pent-up tension, and this area lies on meridians, or energy channels that connect to his pelvis.

You can gain pleasure from having the thyroid glands, located on either side of your throat just under the earlobe, stimulated—all he

TIP

Chakras are energy centers in the body. The "root chakra" is sexual energy that resides at the base of the spine near the anus. So don't ignore it.

needs to do is slowly stroke them with his fingertips to turn you on even more, then run his hands down onto your breasts and nipples, which, of course, have a direct hotline to your clitoris.

More esoterically, if he caresses your wrist bones, this simple act can drive you wild, and also, apparently, it will transmit energy to the heart and increase your emotional passion.

Another good spot for both of you to caress is the "elixir field" (really!), which is the area just above your pubic bone that's very rich in nerve endings. You can both just place your hands there and let the energies course through your bodies—in your case, this should stimulate the G-spot externally and focus your sensations on the area, whereas in his, it's close to his penis so it just feels nice.

Now it gets good. You can experience a labial massage—what one sexpert calls "wibbling." He should simply massage your outer labia—without opening it or entering. He can also caress the inner thighs, creating a circle of stroking. With his fingertips he can "wibble" the soft skin of your labia by pinching it lightly between finger and thumb, but he shouldn't touch your clitoris. I hardly need tell you that this feels nice. And the bonus is, it moves energy around your pelvis, too—you can't lose.

One technique used by Taoists is the "5-minute" technique, whereby you take turns stimulating each other in whatever ways possible for 5 minutes each. After that, you must swap—however desperate you are to continue. If you want built-up sexual energy … well, there's your method.

full body orgasm

Another Eastern philosophy that can have a highly positive effect on your sex life is Taoism. Here, the woman is in control and the point of the slow build-up is a full body orgasm. This is an orgasm that isn't just confined to the genital area—it can suffuse your whole body, traveling around your legs, back up through your stomach and bursting from the top of your head in a shower of sparks, leaving you limp and comatose with post-pleasure exhaustion. Or something like that, at any rate. Some women describe it as a tidal wave they're surfing, while still others find it such an emotional release they end up in tears.

There are various ways to arrive at this marvelous place. Taoism teaches many similar methods to tantra, with a few differences—the

---

TIP

In the early stages of penetration, shallow thrusting is better because it directly stimulates the areas of your vagina that are most sensitive to pressure. When the head of his penis moves back and forth it builds up your excitement. It also means that when he goes in more deeply the upper areas are more ready to respond because you've built up desire. Shallow thrusting also encourages your vagina to contract in an attempt to keep him inside you, which is exciting for him, too. If he then penetrates you deeply, pulls out again, and thrusts shallowly, it creates a vacuum that tugs at the vaginal walls. And guess how good that feels?

> **TIP**
>
> If he massages the hollow between the tendon and the ankle bone, on both sides, it releases blocked kidney energy that leads to sexual inhibition. Massaging here restores lost kidney energy and arouses both of you.

focus is on the genitals, and "vaginal" and "testicular" breathing—I know, I know, but stick with me.

First, release your chi by slapping very lightly on your face, chest and legs—all over, in fact, to awaken your energy channels.

Rotate your hips to get the energy flowing around your body, and make a "shhhh" sound to get rid of tension—come on, it's not that bad, chorus teachers make you do this kind of thing. Well, some do.

The men, meanwhile, are rubbing their perineums (should that be "perinea"?) and pulling on their penises while bending over and sticking their tongues out. Apparently the longer the tongue, the longer the penis, though that may just be something that Taoist teachers say to excuse their pupils from looking like complete fools in front of each other.

Women now need to focus on their "vaginal breathing," which means pulling energy toward their genitals, using deep breathing and concurrent clenching and releasing of the vaginal muscles. Concentrate on your outer labia, and pull inward toward your inner labia, taking a short "sip" of breath with each contraction. Do the same with your anus and perineum for several repetitions. By "breathing" this way you can hold back each time your orgasm seems imminent—take your breath, clench and, as the feeling ebbs and comes back stronger, by the time you finally let it happen you may well have built yourself up to a full body orgasm—don't worry, you'll know if you have.

> **TIP**
>
> To help train your vaginal muscles to the peak of efficiency you can either keep having babies, or do it the easy way. Start by inserting a biggish vibrator and holding that in there—then progress down through cucumbers, bananas, small carrots, finally achieving the muscle control required to hold an object as thin as a pencil. Though if that's his penis, you may have a problem.

Ancient sexual wisdom suggests that the first clitoral orgasm is merely the warm-up act—and that once she's come, she's primed and ready for a more intense vaginal orgasm. The first orgasm dispels fear—just think of how relaxed you feel when you've come—and it allows you to embrace the full sexual experience with your partner afterwards.

Men have an equivalent method—"testicle" breathing relies, again, on him taking his breaths and squeezing his testicles, anus and perineum in a short series of clenches to hold off an orgasm, similar to tantric sex. This method relies on exceptional control and patience from both partners, and if it becomes too difficult, just get the vibrator out.

It is theoretically possible to experience a "spiritual" orgasm from the shared mouth-breathing while you're sitting on his lap with your legs clasped behind him, and his legs crossed so you're as bodily close as it's possible to be. This feels a little like the effects of Reiki healing, which also works on the chakras.

aphrodisiacs

To prepare for your nights of tantric/Taoist lovin', you may want to go the whole way and prepare a feast of aphrodisiacs to get both of you suitably worked up. But don't overeat or you'll end up groaning with indigestion rather than passion. Useful ingredients for your passion-stimulating meal include the following:

- anchovies
- caviar
- honey
- artichokes
- champagne
- salmon
- steak
- ginger
- vanilla

But of course, not all at once, because, without a doubt, you would be sick. Most contain either stamina-boosting or stimulating chemicals—but if you don't want to have an aphrodisiac blow-out, stick with champagne, that's my advice.

yin & yang

The Chinese believe that men and women have different energies—Yin is female, and Yang is male—and that each one has different qualities to bring to life—and sex. Yang energy is dynamic, straightforward and immediate, whereas Yin energy is gentle, receptive and slower-paced. But mingling the two creates a perfect whole, of course. Suggestions for pre-sex mingling of energies—foreplay, in other words—include the reminder that each partner doesn't necessarily want to receive exactly what they're giving because of their different needs and energies. Yang is expected to give appropriately—which may mean responding to her needs very differently than how she responds to his needs. While variety is required in foreplay, the ancient texts make it clear that if there are certain elements of foreplay that your partner loves, it's pointless to cut them out altogether just to be "interesting."

TIP

If you really want to try and come during intercourse, one tip is for him to start by just barely inserting the head of his penis. He goes in and out for a few minutes, then goes in another half-inch, in and out for a few minutes ... keep going, half an inch at a time until he's fully in—at which point you may or may not experience a mind-blowing, earth-shattering orgasm. It takes a lot of restraint for him to manage this, but if he does, it may well pay off big time.

It's also vital to use all of the senses. In Chinese medicine, each sense corresponds to a certain organ—ears with kidneys, tongue with heart, lips with spleen, lungs with nose, and eyes with liver—so stimulating a particular sense helps chi to flow from that organ and theoretically balances your body's energies. Of course, that may strike you as bogus, but the point of the exercise remains—that using all five senses massively enhances your sexual experience. Keep the room light so you can see each other's bodies, and listen to your partner breathing, or gasping, which can be highly erotic. Touch, smell and taste are essential to good sex—scent particularly is the sense most directly connected to our emotional responses (which is why when you smell chalk you're instantly transported back to the classroom with all its attached feelings). Humans secrete pheromones, too, which are chemical "messengers" that arouse the opposite sex, which is why fresh (though not day-old) sweat can be such a turn on.

It's also recommended that you involve your whole body—which isn't as easy as it sounds, since most sexual activity tends to focus on the face, breasts and genitals. Integrating the whole of your bodies invigorates sexual energy in both of you.

oral sex

The spiritual version of oral sex isn't that different from the ordinary version. But much to his delight, it's recommended that you swallow when he comes. Possibly all the writers of ancient Chinese texts were men, but still, as far as they were concerned, semen was a life force that heals all manner of ills (so when your partner insists that it "cures sore throats" he may not be lying quite as much as he thinks he is). In fact, emperors allegedly used to collect the semen of younger men, mix it with herbs, and drink it in a bid to prolong their lives. And they did used to live quite a long time ... but what a price to pay.

Oral sex, however, is considered the second most powerful way of transferring chi between partners—no prizes for guessing the first most powerful. The more chi that flows between you, the more unified you become, and the more strengthened by each other's qualities.

TIP

Some couples find it helpful to designate certain names to their genitals—purely because saying "can you touch me down there," or even "now grab my cock" sounds either clinical or way too porno. The names you choose are entirely down to personal preference, whether calling his penis Mr. Wibbly does it for you, or you actually prefer to use the old "jade stalk" Chinese favorites. He might wish to call your privates "Lady Jane" in the manner of D.H. Lawrence—or he might find "Pussy" works just as well. Whatever you decide, just don't tell anyone else—they're sure to find it nauseating ....

Going down on a man puts him in a more "yin" receptive position, too, and helps him to be more vulnerable and empathetic to the female position. Because the traditional dominant/vulnerable roles are swapped around when you go down on him, you'll have chi flying about like nobody's business—so if it all gets uncomfortable, just give a little, without the pressure of making him come—you can always use your hand instead, or go on to have sex.

Him going down on you—or "drinking from the jade fountain," which sounds a great deal nicer—is also supposed to offer vital health-giving properties. Oral sex is probably the likeliest way a woman will orgasm, too, partly because you can relax without worrying about him and the urgent needs of his jade stalk.

emotional release

Spiritual sex is highly powerful—even if you don't buy into all the chi business. Having this sort of physical and emotional connection with another person opens up dormant areas of feeling, and it's not unusual to burst into tears. If this happens—to you or him—just cuddle each other. You don't need to get into a whole discussion about "oh, I see, now you're in tears, I thought you were having fun ..." unless they genuinely are crying because you had a fight or the boss was a jerk. Otherwise, it's just about unleashing pent-up emotion, so let it happen, and resume what you were doing when everybody calms down.

how to discuss sex

Talking about sex is fraught with problems. Sexuality is such an intimate, vulnerable part of us that actually expressing any negative feelings regarding your or your partner's performance can end in a battle that makes Star Wars look like a playground fight.

It's always easier to discuss sex outside of the bedroom. Once you're halfway through undressing each other, you suddenly piping up, "You know when you do that thing with your mouth? I don't like it," will serve as something of a dampener. Being naked also makes you more vulnerable—so talking with clothes on over a glass of wine one evening places less pressure on you. Don't, however, sit opposite each other at the kitchen table, overhead light glaring down—he'll expect you to state the date and time into a tape recorder before you begin.

Talk around the subject before you get onto it. Talking about intimacy, or how much time you spend together—in, obviously, a non-judgmental and supportive way—can lead naturally onto sex. Whereas saying, "OK, I'm glad you're back. Now, about the way you treat my clitoris," is perhaps not the ideal way to approach it.

When you do get around to it, instigate a discussion about what you like in bed—without ever criticizing things he's done in the past, of course. If that all feels way too confrontational, write him a letter suggesting all the things you could do to each other. Though don't forget to mention things you might do to him.

spiritual intercourse

The positions remain more or less the same—the only difference is in the names. "The dragon turns" sounds better than "missionary," and "treading tigers" is more romantic than "doggy style"—but it still means the same thing. The bit that counts, however, is "transition," from foreplay to intercourse, and for him, suggestions include not always entering you in the same way—sometimes he should thrust in hard,

TIP

While it's fine to go along with a bit of action when you're not really in the mood in the hope that it'll get you going, it's a different thing entirely to be sexually dishonest. If you're faking orgasms, or pretending to enjoy what he's doing when really you're screaming with internal boredom—don't do it. Just tell him the truth, as kindly as you can—and show him what he could be doing differently. Almost everyone wants to make their partner happy and satisfied in bed—so you owe each other the chance to do that. If all it takes is a simple adjustment of the finger or tongue, then surely it's better to find a way of saying so? Communication is the key to satisfying sex—and without it, all the sex tips in the world won't work.

other times tease your clitoris with the tip of his penis before pushing in just a little way. Or he can enter you just two inches or so, then pull out and rub himself on your labia before re-entering. Then he could enter you fast and suddenly, pull back, pause and hover before surprising you by plunging straight back in.

If you're wet enough—or our old pal KY is available—he can enter you very, very slowly—even a centimeter at a time. This feels amazing for him, and builds up your anticipation to a fever pitch. Don't keep it all at this pace, though—you might fall asleep.

He can even enter from a new angle—slightly to one side presses on normally untouched areas of your vaginal wall, and may result in all kinds of excitement. Pulling your vulva apart as he enters is also a new kind of thrill because it exposes your clitoris and the surrounding nerves to much more stimulation than normal.

If he really wants to tease you, he can push at your vaginal entrance—without going any further. After a few pushes, you'll be begging him to enter—and let's face it, he doesn't have that much self control, even if he is a Taoist master ....

Transition suggestions for you include varying the tension of your vaginal muscles, again, by squeezing your PC. Contract as he enters, then release—or vice versa. This is easiest done lying on your back.

Altering the angle of your legs also helps—if you put both feet on one of his shoulders, for example, he can enter you slowly from a new position. Use your hands, too, against his hips, so that you're controlling the depth of penetration—then suddenly move your hips so he thrusts into you at a different angle. Also be aware that sometimes your genitals are arranged in a manner that means they don't fit together perfectly—he might have a long penis and you've got a short vagina, or your clitoris may be too high to be stimulated by his groin when he thrusts. This isn't necessarily a problem but it is worth being aware of because then you can rectify it. If you assume that everyone's built the same you'll feel like it's someone's fault. It isn't—it may just mean you have to find a new way of doing things to ensure your sexual fire burns as brightly as possible for as long as possible.

other books by ulysses press

The Little Bit Naughty Book of Sex
Dr. Jean Rogiere, $9.95

A handy pocket hardcover that is a fun, full-on guide to enjoying great sex.

Secrets of Sexual Body Language
Martin Lloyd-Elliott, $17.95

Shows how to take advantage of the vast world of nonverbal communication by teaching you the basic principles of sending and receiving body language.

Tantra between the Sheets:
The Easy and Fun Guide to Mind-blowing Sex
Val Sampson, $16.00

Removes Tantra from the realm of myth and mystery as it teaches Tantric techniques that enable men and women to feel more sexually confident, become multi-orgasmic and satisfy their lover in the most intimate ways.

The Wild Guide to Sex and Loving
Siobhan Kelly, $16.95

Packed with practical, frank and sometimes downright dirty tips on how to hone your bedroom skills, this handbook tells you everything you need to know to unlock the secrets of truly tantalizing sensual play.

To order these books call 800-377-2542 or 510-601-8301, fax 510-601-8307, e-mail ulysses@ulyssespress.com, or write to Ulysses Press, P.O. Box 3440, Berkeley, CA 94703. All retail orders are shipped free of charge. California residents must include sales tax. Allow two to three weeks for delivery.

P9-BIG-037

The Boxcar Children Mysteries

The Boxcar Children Mysteries

THE MYSTERY OF
THE SOCCER SNITCH

created by
GERTRUDE CHANDLER WARNER

ALBERT WHITMAN & Company
Chicago, Illinois

Library of Congress Cataloging-in-Publication Data

Warner, Gertrude Chandler, 1890-1979.
The mystery of the soccer snitch / created by Gertrude Chandler Warner ;
interior illustrations by Anthony VanArsdale.
pages cm. — (The Boxcar children mysteries ; 136)
Summary: "A talented young soccer player in Greenfield is given the honor of
being a child mascot at an international soccer tournament in Brazil, but when an
anonymous letter insists that she doesn't deserve to go, the Aldens investigate"—
Provided by publisher.
[1. Mystery and detective stories. 2. Soccer—Fiction. 3. Gargoyles—Fiction. 4.
Brothers and sisters—Fiction. 5. Orphans—Fiction.]
I. VanArsdale, Anthony, illustrator. II. Title.
PZ7.W244 2014
[Fic]—dc23
2014002199

THE BOXCAR CHILDREN® is a registered
trademark of Albert Whitman & Company.

10 9 8 7 6 5 4 3 2 1 LB 18 17 16 15 14

Cover art by Logan Kline.
Interior illustrations by Anthony VanArsdale.

For more information about Albert Whitman & Company,
visit our web site at www.albertwhitman.com.

Contents

THE MYSTERY OF
THE SOCCER SNITCH

CHAPTER 1

The Big Day Arrives

"Benny, come on! Hurry!" called Jessie. "The soccer fest starts soon!"

Twelve-year old Jessie was wearing red, her team color.

Benny, who was six and wearing blue, trotted down the stairs. "Will there be lots of food at the soccer feast?"

"Not a soccer *feast*, silly" said Jessie. "A soccer fest!"

"'Fest' means 'festival,'" said Henry, the oldest. "I looked it up." Henry was fourteen and was always looking things up in the dictionary on his new tablet.

"Shouldn't there be food at a festival, then?" Benny asked. "I think there should at least be peanuts and hot dogs and lemonade."

"We had breakfast a half hour ago!" Jessie said. "You ate all those pancakes! You can't be hungry yet."

"I'm not hungry yet," Benny said. "I just think there should be food!"

"The winners get coupons for a free cone at Igloo Ice Cream," Jessie said.

"I sure hope my team wins!" Benny shouted. He didn't see Jessie and Henry exchange smiles. What Jessie and Henry knew—but Benny didn't—was that *all* the children who participated would get a free cone at Igloo Ice Cream.

"Warm ups start soon," Henry said. "We should go."

"This is going to be fun!" Benny said.

"It sure will," Henry said. He was wearing the yellow and black of a referee. All week he'd been studying the referee's manual

Coach Olson had given him. The older boys and girls were assistant coaches and referees.

"Does everyone have their cleats and shin guards?" Henry asked.

"I packed everyone's equipment and an extra ball in this bag," Jessie said. She always brought extra equipment just in case someone needed it.

"Yay!" shouted Benny. "Let's go! Coach Olson said we are all marching in a big parade before the games, just like at the big tournament in Brazil!"

"At the real tournament it's called the opening ceremony," said Henry. "I think in Brazil there will be fireworks."

"I wish we could go to the big tournament!" said Benny. "Kayla is so lucky!"

A few weeks earlier, the town of Greenfield erupted with excitement when the newspaper ran a front-page story with the headline, "Greenfield Girl Chosen as International Child Mascot!" Kayla's parents and Coach Olson quickly organized a soccer fest so everyone could get into the spirit of the upcoming international tournament. The soccer fest would last one day—an opening parade followed by a series of games, ending with an award ceremony—but the children had been practicing for the games almost each day for the past two weeks.

Now, finally, the big day was here.

"We're going to go warm up now, Grandfather!" Jessie called out.

Mr. Alden opened the door to his study. "I'll be along shortly," he said, "before the opening parade."

When Benny opened the front door, Watch, their dog, ran in from the kitchen. Watch panted excitedly, his toenails clipping across the floor.

"Don't worry, Watch," Grandfather told the dog, patting his head. "I'll bring you, too. But you can't go now. The children will be warming up."

After everyone said goodbye, Benny bounded out the door and down the steps to the street. The other three followed.

Together the children walked past

clapboard houses with neat picket fences in front and carefully tended gardens. The sky was clear blue. The air smelled of freshly cut grass and flowers. It was the perfect day for a soccer fest.

Violet felt at ease, walking like this with her brothers and sister. Although they had lost their parents, they had each other, and now, of course, they had Grandfather and Watch.

After their parents died, they ran away because they were afraid of being placed in different homes. They had lived in a boxcar in the woods and entirely took care of themselves—until Grandfather found them, and they learned he was a wonderful person. With him, they could all be together.

Violet was wearing a purple jersey, purple shorts, and lavender socks. She was shy and didn't often raise her hand to speak, but when Coach Olson asked the group of ten-year-old girls what team color they wanted, Violet raised her hand and said purple. Each team also selected the name of a professional team. Violet's team decided to be the purple Wizards.

Getting into the spirit that morning, Violet even laced her cleats with purple shoelaces and tied her pigtails with purple ribbons.

Violet thought about the soccer fest, and parade—and Kayla Thompson. "I wonder if Kayla is excited about being a child mascot in Brazil," she said.

"Kayla has to be excited!" cried Benny. "Why wouldn't she be? Isn't that the whole reason we're having a soccer fest?"

"I don't think she's excited," Violet said. "She doesn't act excited. I understand why. She'll have to go out on the soccer field in front of millions of people."

"I don't think she's shy," Henry said. "She seems very comfortable playing soccer with lots of people watching her."

"That's true," Jessie said. "I think Kayla is just not the type to act excited."

Jessie started to say something more about Kayla, but stopped. She had a vague feeling that Kayla wasn't a very nice person. Other

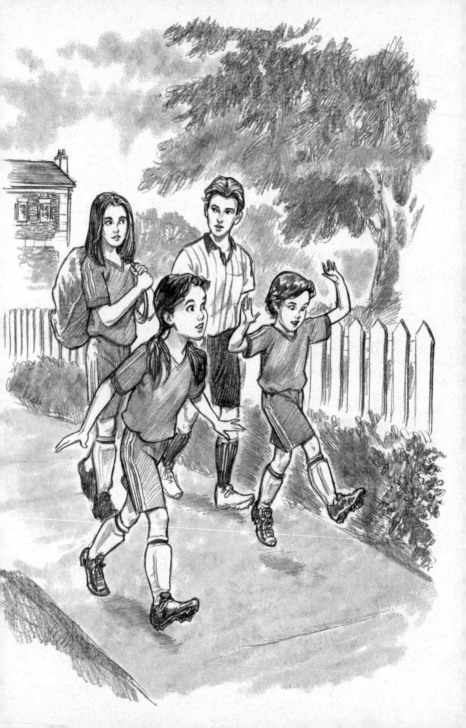

girls in town openly disliked Kayla and even talked badly about her. But, Kayla's family had only recently moved to Greenfield. So nobody really knew Kayla very well. In fact, one girl, Danielle, who was clearly jealous of all the attention Kayla was getting, said Kayla wasn't really a Greenfield girl because she had only lived in the town for six months.

The Alden children arrived at the field to find it decorated with balloons and streamers. The field was large enough for three games to be played at once. Across the street by the playground was another field, also decorated. The streamers—mostly red, white and blue—flapped in the breeze. Each team had a banner with their team color, team name, and the name of each player.

"There's my team!" Benny shouted. "The Earthquakes!"

The players gathered with their teams to the side of the field and did warm-up exercises. First they practiced dribbling, then they practiced passing the ball to each other.

Toward the end of their warm-up exercises,

the bleachers filled with spectators. Jessie looked over and saw Grandfather taking a seat in the bleachers. Next to him was Mrs. McGregor, his housekeeper, and several of his friends. Watch lay on the ground nearby, panting because of the heat. This time of year—late August, just after school started— always seemed like the hottest time of year.

Coach Olson blew his whistle and the teams ran to the side of the field. The high school marching band was already in formation.

Benny was jumping with excitement. All around him, small children were jumping and wiggling and good-naturedly pushing each other, eager to get started.

Jessie, watching him, smiled. Her team, all dressed in red, had chosen the name Chicago Fire.

Coach Olson blew his whistle, and the marching band marched onto the field. The drums rolled, *rat-a-tat-tat*, *rat-a-tat-tat*. The crowd cheered and clapped and stamped their feet. The band played "My Country 'Tis of Thee," a song Jessie always found stirring.

Next came the high school majorettes in their sequined uniforms twirling and tossing their batons. The batons glittered in the sun.

The first team to march onto the field was Jessie's team, the Chicago Fire. Leading the team was Kayla, dribbling a ball and performing fancy footwork. She did a fake, pretending she was going to pass the ball and instead stepping on it and pushing it behind her. Next she kicked the ball, causing it to fly straight up, then she bounced it twice on her shoulders. She stepped back and the ball landed directly at her feet and she began dribbling again.

I wish I could do that, Jessie thought.

The audience, many of whom had never seen Kayla's skills, shouted "oooh!" and "aaah!"

"She's just a show-off," said Danielle, one of Jessie's teammates who made no secret of her dislike for Kayla.

"Shh," whispered Jessie.

After the teams circled the field, the marching band played "Yankee Doodle

Dandy." When the last of the drums quieted, Coach Olson walked up to a small wooden platform.

He picked up his microphone. He turned it on, and it made a brief screeching sound. He cleared his throat and said, "Welcome! Welcome to the first Greenfield Soccer Fest!" His voice boomed across the field.

Everyone cheered. Jessie looked over at Grandfather and smiled. He smiled back.

"The players have been working hard," said the coach, "practicing and preparing, getting ready for today's grand tournament. Each team will play three games—"

"Stop everything!" came a shout. Mrs. Thompson, Kayla's mother, was marching angrily toward the field, holding her cell phone. "Stop everything right now!"

Everyone fell silent. Jessie could see right away that Mrs. Thompson was angry. Her face was red, her frown deep.

"What is going on?" Coach Olson asked.

Mrs. Thompson marched to the foot of the platform. "Somebody in this town has written a letter to the mascot committee! A letter filled with horrible lies about Kayla. I just received a phone call from the committee. Now she might not get to be mascot!"

Coach Olson hadn't turned off the microphone, so Mrs. Thompson's voice carried over the entire field.

When Coach Olson flipped off the microphone, there was a screech of static, then more silence.

Jessie and the other girls on the red team turned to look at Kayla.

Kayla held perfectly still for a long moment, then buried her face in her hands.

CHAPTER 2

A Horrible Letter

Mrs. Thompson walked briskly across the field toward the red team. The coach jumped down from the platform and hurried to catch up to her. Upon reaching the girls, Mrs. Thompson touched Kayla's shoulder to comfort her. Mrs. Thompson didn't look at the other girls. Jessie still felt too astonished to speak, or even move.

"Who would do such a thing?" asked the coach, approaching.

"That's just it!" Mrs. Thompson said. "We

13

don't know! Whoever wrote the letter didn't sign it. But now the mascot committee wants Kayla investigated, just to make sure the things in the letter are not true."

Kayla whirled around and, keeping her face hidden, ran from the soccer field. She ran past her mother, down the street toward her home.

Then everyone, it seemed, started talking at once.

"I wonder what is in the letter!"

"I wonder who wrote it!"

"I wonder what will happen now!"

The coach and Mrs. Thompson stepped aside and whispered together. As they talked, Mrs. Thompson made angry gestures, hitting her fist into her palm and pointing toward the field.

Danielle, standing not far from Jessie but out of Mrs. Thompson's earshot, whispered, "I don't think Kayla deserved to be mascot anyway. The mascot should be someone nice, not someone who just shows off."

"I am so tired of listening to you talk mean

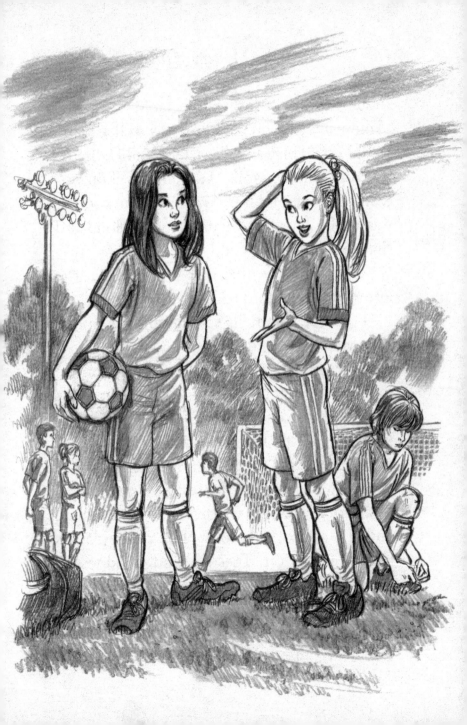

about Kayla," another girl told Danielle. "You just wish you could play as well as her."

"If I could play as well as her," said Danielle, twirling her ponytail, "I'd be nicer about it." Danielle had a long ponytail reaching to her waist. Her hair was very thick and blond and she was obviously proud of it.

"Maybe *you're* the one who wrote the letter," Jennifer said to Danielle.

"I did not," Danielle said, flipping her pony tail over her shoulder.

A few parents from the bleachers went to join Mrs. Thompson and Coach Olson. The parents and Coach Olson talked for several moments. Then Coach Olson strode back to the podium and turned on his microphone.

"We will continue the fest next Saturday!" he announced. "We will have the games then, and the award ceremony. The older players will practice on Tuesday and Wednesday after school, as usual. The younger players—the Earthquakes and Galaxies—can practice tomorrow at one o'clock. We should have this all sorted out by next Saturday."

Nobody in the stands moved. A slight breeze moved in the trees. From the distance came the barking of a dog. Otherwise, all was quiet.

Henry, Jessie, Violet, and Benny looked for each other, and huddled in a group.

"We need to figure out who wrote the letter," Henry whispered to his sisters and brother.

"Yes," Jessie said. "This isn't fair at all."

"I wonder if we can see the letter!" said Benny. "Do you think Mrs. Thompson has it?"

"She said she got a phone call from the mascot committee," Jessie said. "So the committee probably has it."

"That's too bad," said Henry. "If we could see the letter, we could examine the postmark and see how it was written."

"I wonder who did it," Jessie said. She was looking toward Danielle.

"Do you think it was Danielle?" Violet asked.

"Actually," Jessie said, "it could have been

any of the girls on the team, not just the ones who speak up and say they don't like Kayla. The problem is, I don't know anyone on the team who would make up lies."

"Lying is bad," Benny said.

"Lying in a letter to get someone in trouble is even worse," Henry said.

Violet looked over the group of girls wearing red. There were at least a dozen of them. "We've never started out with this many suspects before," she said.

All four of the Alden children stood still for a moment, thinking this over.

"Here comes Grandfather and Mrs. McGregor and Watch!" Benny said. Benny ran toward them. The others followed behind. Watch greeted each of the children with a sniff and wag of his tail. Benny petted Watch's back while Henry scratched the top of Watch's head.

Mr. Alden said, "Well, children, I suppose we should head home."

"I was hoping to win a cone from Igloo Ice Cream," Benny said.

"Maybe next week," Henry said.

They headed down the sidewalk. Mr. Alden took a handkerchief from his pocket and patted his forehead. "It's going to be a hot day today," he said.

"The forecast is calling for high temperatures all week," Mrs. McGregor said.

"What are we going to do today?" Benny asked. "We thought we'd be here all day!"

"Mr. Beck is working at the house," Mrs. McGregor said. "So I suppose we can start by seeing how he's doing." Mr. Beck was the handyman Mr. Alden hired when they needed work done on the house.

"And," Mrs. McGregor said, "it looks to me like you children have a mystery to solve."

Violet sighed deeply. "Poor Kayla. I feel so sorry for her."

"Me, too," Henry said. "I don't know which is worse, not getting to be an international child mascot, or knowing someone wrote a mean letter filled with lies."

"At least it shouldn't be too hard to prove that the letter was filled with the lies," Jessie said. "Then Kayla can still be the mascot."

The first thing Violet noticed as they walked up the front walk to their house was the smell of saw dust. She and the others walked around to the side of the house. Mr. Beck was up on a ladder scooping leaves out of the gutter.

"What are you doing?" Benny asked.

"Routine summer stuff," Mr. Beck said. "I just replaced some rotted boards in the garage. Now I'm cleaning the gutters. Next I'll check the windows. You have to watch out with these old windows in the summer." He squinted up at the roof line. "And it looks like a few roof tiles are loose. I'd better fix those."

"Can I help you?" Benny asked. "I can climb the ladder, too!"

"Better not, Benny," said Mr. Alden. "I think Mr. Beck can manage just fine."

"All right," Benny said. "Let's go have a snack! I can solve mysteries better with a full stomach!"

CHAPTER 3

A Not-Quite-So-Horrible Letter

Henry was the first one at the breakfast table the next morning. While waiting for the others, he'd opened the newspaper. Ordinarily Henry read the news on his tablet, but the local Greenfield newspaper had not gone digital yet. Grandfather was happy about that. He said he liked a real newspaper over breakfast and before bed.

"Would you all come look at this?" Henry called. "Amazing!"

Jessie and Violet came running from the

kitchen. "What?" Jessie asked.

"Here's a copy of the letter to the Mascot Committee! It says here that the letter was written in the library computer lab. A reporter found a copy in the automatic save file and printed it here!"

"What does the letter say?" Violet asked.

Henry, Violet, and Jessie leaned over the table and read:

Dear Members of the Mascot Committee,
This letter is to tell you all the reasons Kayla Thompson should not be an international mascot. The mascot should be someone who is a team player and who gives soccer a good name. Kayla is not a team player. She hogs the ball. She laughs when other people make mistakes. She shows off. She is not friendly and people don't like her. For all these reasons, she should not be a child mascot.
Yours sincerely,
Concerned citizens of Greenfield, Connecticut.

All three children finished reading at the same time. They lifted their heads and looked at each other.

"But," Henry said, "some of those things aren't lies."

"Most of these things aren't lies," Jessie said, "Everything here is sort of true."

"But wait," Violet said, "isn't some of that a matter of opinion? Different people can have different opinions about whether she's friendly."

"The fact is," Jessie said, "she's not a team player. She does hog the ball."

"Does she laugh when people make mistakes?" Henry asked.

"I've never seen her laugh," Jessie said. "She's usually concentrating on what she's doing, not paying much attention to anyone else."

Just then, Benny came bounding down the stairs. "What were you hollering about, Henry?"

Before Henry could answer, Grandfather came in from his study and Mrs. McGregor brought a pitcher of fresh milk and a plate of French toast.

"My favorite!" Benny said. "French toast! With syrup!"

"I was just coming to help with breakfast," Jessie told Mrs. McGregor, "but I got so distracted by the news about Kayla!"

"What news about Kayla?" Mrs. McGregor asked.

"How about if we all sit down and talk about the news over breakfast," Mr. Alden said.

The children, Mr. Alden, and Mrs. McGregor sat at the table. Mrs. McGregor passed around a plate of French toast. When it was Benny's turn, he carefully selected the largest piece. Then he looked up and said, "Does anyone mind?"

"Go ahead, Benny," Grandfather said with an indulgent smile.

Henry poured himself a glass of orange juice, then said, "The newspaper ran a copy of the letter someone wrote to the International Mascot Committee about Kayla."

"What did the letter say?" Benny asked.

"Here," Henry said, handing him the newspaper. "You can read it yourself."

Benny squinted at the newspaper. "But I'm

eating! Read it aloud. Please!"

"Yes, please do," Grandfather said. "Then we can all hear it."

Henry read the letter aloud. When he finished, Grandfather said, "Well, that's very interesting. What do you children think?"

"I think it sounds just like what girls like Danielle are always saying about Kayla," Jessie said. "And none of those things are really lies."

"That's why we have so many suspects," Violet told Mr. Alden. "So many girls don't like Kayla. It could have been any of them."

"You know," Henry said. "I don't think writing a letter with things that are true is something a person can get in trouble for."

"But it wasn't very nice," Violet said.

"Oh I agree with that," Henry said. "It wasn't nice. But it isn't what we thought at first. And it isn't what Mrs. Thompson said. Nobody wrote a letter with lies. They wrote a letter with the truth. That's different."

"I don't think it's fair for an anonymous letter to ruin a person's chance to do something as exciting as being an international mascot," Jessie said.

"If someone didn't like Kayla," Benny said, "she should have talked to Kayla or gotten a grown-up to help."

"Exactly," Violet said. "Writing that letter was mean. Whoever wrote it should work things out with Kayla and leave the Mascot Committee out of it."

Tap, tap, tap. Everyone looked up, startled.

"What was that?" Benny asked.

"Sounds like someone is hammering outside!" Jessie said.

"Let's go see!" Benny leapt to his feet and ran to the back door. The others followed.

Outside they found Mr. Beck on the ladder again, tapping at the wood trim around the window with his hammer.

"It's Sunday!" Mrs. McGregor exclaimed. "What on earth are you doing up there?"

"Just finishing up," he said. "It's going to be so hot this week, I wanted to get the last of the work finished up this morning."

"It's hard to believe it can get hotter than

this," Henry said, wiping his brow.

"It can," Mr. Beck said, "and according to the weather report, it will."

***

Later that day, Henry told Benny, "Get ready! It almost time for your practice!"

Benny had been playing with toy cars on the living room floor. He jumped up and ran to his room to change clothes. Henry, who helped coach the youngest children, was already ready.

"I'd come with you to watch for clues," Jessie said, "but it's so hot out there!"

Jessie and Violet were at a table in the living room. Jessie was reading a book, Violet was drawing in her sketchpad.

"No need!" Henry said. "Benny and I will watch for clues."

***

Nothing unusual happened during Benny's practice—until the very end, when the players were practicing dribbling down the field. Coach Olson was watching them, shouting out reminders to watch where they were going and touch the ball with the insides of their shoes instead of the tips of their toes. Henry looked over and saw Mrs. Thompson approaching.

The coach saw her too. He said, "Henry, take over. It looks like I need to speak to Mrs. Thompson."

Henry wished he could move closer to Mrs. Thompson and the coach to hear what they were saying, but he had no choice. He had to keep reminding the players to watch were they were going. If they were not constantly reminded to keep their eyes up, they watched their feet instead of where they were doing, sometimes crashing into each other.

Whenever Henry had the chance to look over at Coach Olson and Mrs. Thompson, he could see she seemed angry at the coach. Coach Olson seemed to cower away from her.

After they spoke a few minutes and Mrs. Thompson left, the coach blew his whistle. "Everyone take a water break!" he shouted.

Some children ran for their water bottles. Others ran for the fountain.

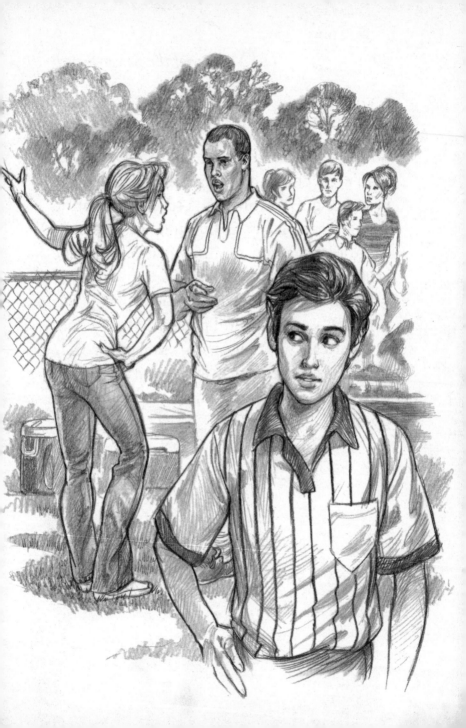

"She seemed angry," Henry said to the coach.

"She is," Coach Olson said. "She thinks I didn't react quickly enough and that I am not protecting Kayla. She thinks the investigation should have taken an hour and not a week."

"I don't see how an investigation can take just one hour," Henry said.

"I don't either," Coach Olson replied.

"She's a very forceful person," Henry said.

"You can say that again," said the coach. "There is something fishy about this whole thing. I don't know what, but something doesn't seem right."

CHAPTER 4

Captain of the Team

When Jessie arrived for practice Tuesday, several of the girls, including Kayla, were already there. Kayla was dribbling down field. The other girls, as usual, were trying to get the ball away from her. The first thing Jessie noticed was that Kayla was smiling. It wasn't a big, happy smile. Kayla just wasn't the type to wear big happy smiles. But she was smiling. Her face was bright.

Then Kayla turned and passed the ball to Samantha. That was different! Kayla rarely passed the ball to anyone. Jessie understood why Kayla rarely passed the ball. The other girls often fumbled and lost the ball. Kayla knew she could do better if she kept the ball to herself.

"Nice work, Kayla and Samantha!" shouted Mia.

Mia was the fifteen-year-old girl who was helping coach Jessie's team.

Jessie felt eager and hopeful. Perhaps everything was resolved. Why else would Kayla suddenly be behaving differently? Perhaps the letter writer stepped forward, apologized and took everything back, and the investigation was over. Perhaps, too, Kayla learned her lesson and would be nicer now when she played. Jessie hoped so.

Jessie put on her shin guards, and changed from her sneakers to her cleats. She took the extra balls from her bag and brought them to the field.

Betsy, one of Jessie's friends, ran up and said, "Hi there, Jess!" Betsy also seemed to be smiling. Nobody would have known, from how all the girls were behaving, that a scandal recently rocked the town.

"Hi," Jessie said. "Everyone looks so happy. Is anything new?"

"Nothing is new. Kayla got here early. She's acting different. Much nicer. C'mon. Let's play!"

Betsy ran to join the girls, who were then down field taking turns kicking the ball into the goal. Jessie followed. Just then, Kayla passed the ball to another teammate so the other girl could practice scoring.

"See," Betsy said quietly to Jessie. "She's acting different. She's being more of a team player."

"She probably wants to show that the things in the letter aren't true," Jessie said.

"But everyone knows they *are* true!" Betsy said, and darted away.

Jessie followed. She was thinking people can change. Wouldn't it be nice if the letter ended up helping Kayla see her bad behavior? Jessie smiled at her own thoughts. Usually Violet was the optimistic one.

"Whew, it's hot!" Danielle called out. "I need more water!" She ran to the side of the field for her water bottle.

"Just pour the water right on your head!" advised Lara. "I did that and I feel great!'

Lara, indeed, was dripping with water. Danielle laughed and poured water on her own head. She also poured water on her long pony tail. Then several other girls, including Jessie, did the same. Jessie laughed. She felt much cooler.

After they'd been practicing a half hour, Mia said, "It's so hot, I think we should stop early."

The girls standing nearby agreed.

Jessie went to drink some more water. Some of the girls gathered to the side of the field, not far from her. That was when Jessie heard Danielle talking quietly to Ashley. "What's happening with the investigation? Did anyone find out who wrote that letter?"

"The coach is investigating. Didn't he talk to you yet?"

"No," Danielle said.

"He talked to me," Ashley said. "I think he's talking to everyone. You'll get a turn. Then you can tell him what you think of Kayla."

Jessie turned away, disappointed. She had hoped the problems had been resolved. She sighed. She supposed the coach would talk to her, too. When it was her turn, she would tell him she didn't think it fair for Kayla to get punished because of an anonymous letter.

"Gather around!" Mia called. "The coach says all the teams need to select a captain. He says we should have done that in the first place. So does anyone want to nominate someone?"

Jessie raised her hand. "I nominate Kayla. She is the best player. I like how she played today, during practice."

"All right," Mia said. "Kayla is nominated. Any other nominations?"

"I nominate Jessie," Betsy said. "Jessie is a good player, too."

Other girls nodded in agreement. Jessie was the second best player on the team.

"Any other nominations?" Mia asked.

"I nominate Danielle," Ashley said.

"Anyone else?" Mia asked.

Nobody said anything.

"Okay," Mia said. "We have three nominations. That should be good enough." She handed everyone a piece of paper and passed around pencils. "The votes will be secret. Everyone can write one name."

After everyone finished writing, Mia collected the pieces of paper. She went to sit by herself to count the votes. She came back and said, "Jessie wins. Jessie is the team captain."

The girls nearby turned to congratulate Jessie.

"Being team captain is a big responsibility," Mia said. "The team captain looks out for everyone. If you aren't sure what to do in the middle of the game, look at Jessie. She'll make the decisions."

Betsy leaned close to Jessie and whispered, "You'll be great!"

"Thanks," Jessie whispered back. She felt

flattered—and sorry for Kayla. She believed Kayla should have been team captain. After all, Kayla was the best player.

"Let's meet back here at the same time tomorrow," Mia called out. "Don't forget to bring a water bottle! Tomorrow is supposed to be even hotter." Then Mia turned to Jessie and said, "Coach Olson wants to know if Henry can help me coach your team tomorrow. Coach Olson said he's a really good coach."

"I'll ask him," Jessie said, "but I'm sure he can."

Jessie removed her shin guards and changed from her cleats to her sneakers. She was walking home when she saw Kayla, by herself, sitting on a bench by the playground, tying her shoe laces.

Jessie approached her. With a friendly smile, she said, "Hello."

Kayla glanced at Jessie. "Hello," she responded. Her eyebrows went into a high arch, and there was a surprised lilt to her voice. Obviously she wasn't used to people being friendly to her.

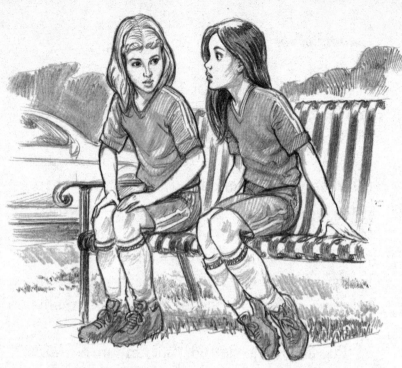

Jessie decided it was best just to come right out and say what nobody wanted to say. "I saw that letter in the paper. I thought it was terrible, and very unfair."

Kayla grimaced. It was almost as if a dark cloud passed over her face. Instantly Jessie regretted her words. She should have realized the whole subject would be painful for Kayla. She hadn't intended to cause Kayla more pain. She just wanted to be friendly.

"Thanks," Kayla said. She stood up and picked up her soccer bag. "I think I'll go now."

Just before leaving, Kayla said, "Thanks for nominating me. And congratulations on being elected team captain."

"It should have been you," Jessie said.

Kayla gave a sad, wistful smile, then waved and walked away.

***

At the dinner table that evening, Jessie told Henry that the coach wanted to know if he'd help coach her team. "Of course," said Henry. "Helping Mia will be fun."

"Did anything interesting happen at your practice?" Benny asked.

"Well, the team elected me captain," Jessie said.

"Congratulations!" Grandfather said. "That's an honor! It means your teammates respect you and look to you as a leader."

"I think Kayla should have been captain," Jessie said.

"The captain isn't always the best player," Henry said. "The captain is the best team player, the one who looks out for everyone else and chooses which plays the team should do."

"I will tell you this," Jessie said. "If Danielle or Ashley wrote the letter, they're clever about pretending they didn't. Danielle and Ashley talked about the letter as if they didn't write it, and didn't know who did."

"You'd think whoever wrote the letter would have known about the automatic save function at the library," Henry said.

"The what?" Benny asked.

"Kids were always losing their homework when they forgot to save their work," Henry said. "So now there is an automatic save. Don't you remember? That's how the reporter found the copy."

"So whoever wrote the letter doesn't know about the autosave?" Jessie asked. "I wonder if there are any clues in that."

"I think all the older kids know about autosave," Henry said. "And the teachers know."

"Maybe it wasn't one of the kids or teachers," Benny said. "Maybe it was a grown-up in town who doesn't like the Thompsons."

"Well, Benny," Henry said. "How about if tomorrow before Jessie's practice you and I visit the library and see if we can find out if anyone other than teachers or students were using the computers."

"Good idea!" Benny said.

***

The next day, at school, Jessie was in the school library during her study period when she felt a gentle tap on her shoulder. She turned. There was Coach Olson, smiling.

"May I speak to you for a few minutes," he asked.

"Of course!" Jessie said.

Jessie and Coach Olson sat at the table in the library conference room. Coach Olson had an open friendly face and an easy smile.

"You probably know why I want to talk to you," he said. "I am investigating the accusations in the letter. The mascot committee wants to know whether they are true."

"You should have seen how nice Kayla was at the practice yesterday!" Jessie said. "She passed the ball to other girls so they could score, too. She was friendly, and a team player."

"But she generally isn't a team player, right? Ordinarily, she does not show team spirit. Do you agree with that?"

Jessie looked down into her lap. She understood why Mrs. Thompson was not happy with the coach, since it was clear he didn't like Kayla, and didn't think she should be mascot.

"Kayla is the best player on the team," Jessie said. "By far. I think she can learn to be a team player, if someone helps her."

The coach smiled at her and said, "You are very supportive of your teammates. All of them. Mia said that's why you were elected team captain."

Jessie felt confused, wondering why he was suddenly talking about her.

"Thank you," she said.

***

The downtown library was crowded after school. "I'll bet everyone wants to be in here where it's nice and cool," Benny whispered to Henry.

Henry agreed. All the comfortable reading

chairs were taken. The carpet in the picture book room was also filled with children sprawled out, reading. Henry and Benny walked to the back of the library where the row of computers were lined up on a table against the back wall. A few kids were doing homework. Several of the computers were empty. Benny and Henry sat down and looked around.

One of the librarians came to them and said, "Can I help you boys with anything?"

"We were curious about that letter the reporter found," Henry said.

"Very clever of that reporter," said the librarian. "She came in and asked if the computers had automatic save functions. I said they did, and she said she wanted to look for something. She spent about twenty minutes looking through one homework assignment after another. Then she found the letter."

"I only see students using the computers," Henry said. "And sometimes teachers."

"Mostly students," said the librarian. "But

occasionally we get adults, too, who are not connected to the school."

"Do you need a library card to use the computers?" Benny asked.

"Nope, anyone can use them. We charge for printing, but anyone can print."

A boy sitting at a computer nearby raised his hand for help. The librarian excused herself and went to help him.

Benny and Henry looked at each other.

"The letter was typed, so there are no clues in the handwriting," Benny said.

"And the postmark probably shows that it was mailed from the Greenfield post office. No clues there."

"I don't think we learned anything helpful," Benny said.

"I don't think so, either," Henry said with a sigh.

CHAPTER 5

Danielle Does Something Mean

Wednesday was the hottest day yet. The air was so humid that simply walking across the street was enough to make a person feel groggy, hot, and tired. Some of the teams cancelled their practice, but the red team decided to practice anyway, even though it seemed to Jessie that the heat was making everyone feel a little cross.

When Jessie and Henry approached the field, Mia called out, "I'm so glad you could come help, Henry!"

The field was freshly mowed, so the air smelled of cut grass. Ordinarily the smell of cut grass was one of Jessie's favorite smells because it reminded her of summer. But today, the smell seemed too heavy and sweet. She was so hot she felt wet all over.

It was Jessie's turn to be the goalie. She stood waiting in front of the goal while Danielle dribbled the ball toward her. Just when it looked as if Danielle would easily kick the ball into the goal, Kayla darted in front of her, as if from nowhere, and with a single kick, took the ball away from her. In a flash, Kayla was dribbling in the other direction.

"Show-off!" Danielle said, flipping her long pony tail over her shoulder.

"I'm not showing off," Kayla said. "I'm playing soccer the way you're supposed to play soccer."

"You're always showing off," Danielle said.

"You're always being mean," Kayla retorted. "You and your mean friends."

Betsy said to Danielle, "You just don't like

that Kayla can get the ball away from you so easily."

Danielle turned away, but not before Jessie saw the angry look that crossed her face. Jessie braced herself, waiting for Danielle to say something else mean. But Danielle didn't say anything. She put both hands in the pockets of her shorts. Jessie thought that was odd.

A few minutes later, Henry blew his whistle and called out to Danielle, "Why are you running with your hands in your pockets?"

Danielle ignored him. She kept her hands in her pockets.

Henry and Jessie exchanged puzzled glances. "We'd better keep an eye on them," Jessie said.

"Oh, yes," Henry said.

"Can someone else have a turn being goalie now?" Jessie asked. The goalie has to stay near the goal. Jessie wanted to stay close to Danielle and Kayla.

"Certainly," Mia said, "if you don't want to any more."

"How about Jennifer?" Jessie suggested. "She hasn't had a turn yet."

Jessie took off the goalie's vest and threw it to Jennifer. As the girls ran up and down the field, practicing, Jessie made sure to stay between Danielle and Kayla. She wanted to be able to prevent trouble, if she could. She knew from the way Kayla and Danielle looked at each other that both of them were still angry.

Ashley was dribbling toward the goal. Kayla easily stole the ball from her, then turned and dribbled the opposite direction.

Just then, in a flash, Danielle darted in front of Kayla. She took something from her pocket and dropped it on the ground at Kayla's feet.

Kayla tripped. She screamed and sprawled forward. She landed face down, in the grass.

Jessie ran to Kayla, and knelt next to her. "Kayla! Are you okay?"

Kayla pushed herself up to a sitting position. She had grass stuck to the side of her jersey and some mud on her face.

Others, including Henry, ran over and knelt next to Kayla.

"I'm fine," Kayla said. Jessie could see she was shaky and angry. Mia ran to them. Together, Jessie and Mia helped Kayla to her feet.

Kayla looked down to see what she'd tripped on. There, on the ground at her feet, was a golf ball. Kayla picked up the golf ball, and marched over to Danielle. "Did you do this?"

Jessie ran to be next to Kayla. "It's okay, Kayla," Jessie said. "Let's not have a fight."

Kayla shook the golf ball at Danielle. For a horrible moment, Jessie thought Kayla was going to throw it at her. Instead, Kayla whirled around and said, "I'm finished."

Kayla dropped the ball into her own pocket. She went to the bench, picked up her water bottle and sports bag, and walked from the field. The other girls were silent, watching, as she crossed the street and sat on a bench. She changed from her cleats into her regular shoes.

"Maybe we should stop for today," Mia said. "Everyone is a little testy."

"You can say that again!" one of the girls said.

"I'm glad she won't be mascot," Ashley said.

Jessie shot Ashley a quick glance. She couldn't understand how anyone could take sides against the girl who had just been tripped. Jessie looked closely at Ashley. Maybe Ashley and Danielle were the ones who had written that letter to sabotage Kayla's chances.

"My opinion," Mia said, "is that Jessie should be mascot."

"I don't want to be mascot," Jessie said quickly. "I wouldn't want to take something away from someone else like that."

"But you're the kind of player who *should* be mascot," Mia said.

The girls sat on benches to change into their sneakers. Jessie put her shin guards and the extra balls she had brought into her soccer bag and slung the bag over her shoulder.

Henry and Jessie walked home together. It seemed to Jessie that the entire town was moving in slow motion because of the heat. There were not many cars on the street, and only a few people on the sidewalk.

"Mrs. McGregor asked if we can stop at the market for some milk," Henry said. "That's why I brought this." He pointed to the backpack he was wearing.

"All right," Jessie said.

They turned a corner toward the market and there, in front of them, was Kayla, heading toward her house. Kayla's hands were in her pockets.

"You sure are right about those girls," Henry said. "They can be mean."

"Yes, they can," Jessie agreed. "Ever since Kayla came to the school, the girls have been mean to her."

Kayla was walking faster than Henry and Jessie, so soon she was at the corner, ready to cross the street. Idly, as Henry and Jessie watched, Kayla took the golf ball from her pocket, looked at it, and rubbed it against

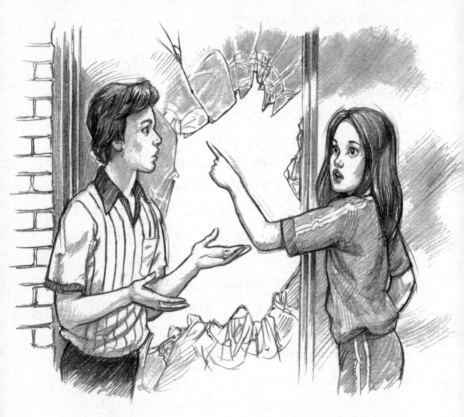

her shirt the way a person might brush off an apple before eating it. Then she dropped it back into her pocket. She turned the corner and was gone from their sight.

Henry and Jessie turned the corner toward the market. Henry looked down an alley where Gerry's General Store used to be. The sign still said, "Gerry's General Store," even though Gerry had closed his store and moved from town over the winter. There was a "For Lease" sign in the window.

"Would you look at that!" Henry said. "The window is broken!"

Jessie peered down the street. "It is!" she said. At first she hadn't noticed because the storefront was in shadows.

"I wonder when that happened," Henry said. "I didn't notice it this morning. We should tell Grandfather so he can let the police know."

"Maybe we should look," said Jessie, "to make sure nothing was left dangerous."

Henry and Jessie quickly walked down the alley to the store. Glass was everywhere. The wood casing was splintered.

Just then a door opened and Mrs. Leob, a friend of Grandfather's, came out of a nearby shop. Seeing the broken glass, she shrieked. She turned to Henry and Jessie, "Did you do this?"

"No, ma'am, we did not!" Henry said. "We saw the broken glass and came over to look."

Mrs. Leob looked closely at Henry and Jessie. "Oh! You're the Alden children! I was so upset I didn't notice! Did you see anything suspicious?"

"No, ma'am," Henry said.

"I will call the police right away," Mrs. Leob said. "We do not put up with this sort of behavior in Greenfield. Whoever did this will find himself—or herself—in big, big trouble."

Just then, Jessie noticed something else. Cold air was coming from the inside of the store. "It seems like an air conditioner is on in there," Jessie said.

"You're right!" Henry said. "The air is freezing! How odd!"

"What a waste of energy," Mrs. Leob said. "I will have the police turn it off when they get here."

CHAPTER 6

A Friend in the Woods

Meanwhile, Violet was at home. The purple team didn't practice that day. Their coaches—two eighth-grade girls—said it was simply too hot. So Violet did her homework, then sat in the living room with her sketch pad. She was in an after school art class which met once weekly, on Mondays. Grandfather bought her a new sketchpad for the class. Already she'd filled most of her sketchpad with lovely drawings.

She pulled a chair to the window. From

the chair, she could see the flowerbeds in the front yard. She drew the rosebushes. She liked drawing nature—trees, flowers, birds. After filling a few pages with drawings of the flowerbed, she went to Grandfather's study. His door was open and he was at his writing desk, working. She tapped softly on the door frame.

He looked up.

"Grandfather, may I take my sketch book into the woods so I can draw some trees and wild flowers."

"Certainly," he said. "Take some water with you to drink. And don't forget to be back by dinner time."

She walked from the house, down the street to the trail leading into the woods. A short distance into the woods, she found a cool glade. She spread a blanket in the shade and settled down with her sketch pad and drawing pencils. There, in a sunny spot, was a patch of beautiful pink flowers with five soft petals and a yellow center. She knew the names of the flower from a book she'd read in school the year before. The flowers were called pasture roses, but they didn't look anything like garden roses. They had a simple shape, just five petals, so they were easy to draw.

Soon she filled her sketchbook page with pasture roses. She was drawing grass to frame the picture when she heard the crunching of footsteps through the woods. The person was coming from the opposite direction Violet had come, so she suspected whoever was approaching was not her sister or one of her brothers.

She looked up and waited.

To her surprise, from around the corner, came Kayla, carrying a sketch pad. Kayla stopped, obviously surprised to see Violet. The two girls looked at each other for a moment.

Kayla said, "Sorry," and turned to leave.

"You can stay," Violet said. "This is a nice place to draw."

Kayla hesitated. Violet noticed Kayla had a serious sort of face. Her lips were thin and a bit pale, her eyebrows were light, her eyes a cool gray-blue. She didn't seem like the kind of girl who smiled much.

Violet made room on her blanket. Kayla sat down and took out a sharpened pencil and began to sketch a nearby tree.

Violet tried not to watch. She tried to concentrate on her own picture. But Kayla was sitting close enough so Violet couldn't help but see what Kayla was drawing.

"That's really good," Violet said. Violet wasn't just being nice. Kayla's picture was good. Kayla sketched with light, soft touches of her pencil, perfectly capturing the rough texture of the bark and the shape of the trunk.

"So is yours," Kayla said.

"I like to draw," Violet said.

"Me, too," Kayla said.

Violet returned to her drawing, deeply surprised. Kayla was nothing at all like she expected. She'd had the feeling all along that people were wrong about Kayla. Now she knew for sure that people were misjudging her.

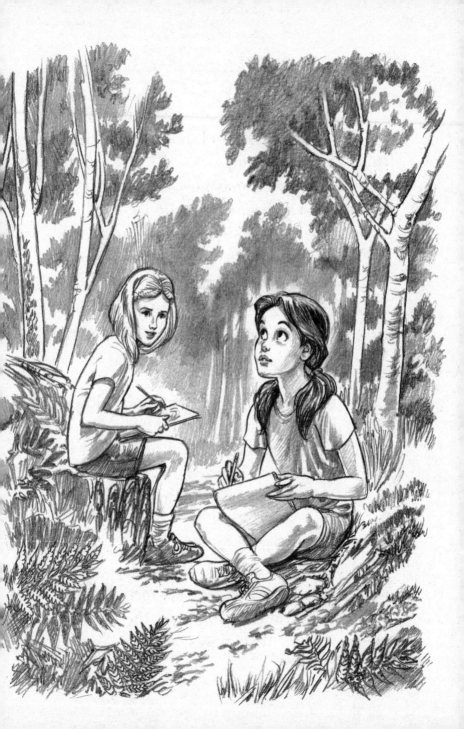

The girls sat quietly, drawing, until Violet noticed, from the slant of the sun, that dinner time was approaching.

"I should go home now," she said. "I'm supposed to be back before dinner."

"Me, too," said Kayla, standing up.

Kayla helped Violet fold up her blanket. Just before Kayla turned to go, she said, "Thank you for not saying anything about you-know-what. I am tired of talking about it."

"I understand," Violet said.

"Even when people are being nice, I don't like talking about it."

"I understand," Violet said again. And she did. Violet didn't like to talk much either, particularly to people she didn't know well.

***

When the Aldens were sitting at the dinner table, eating, Violet said, "I saw Kayla in the woods today. She seemed very nice."

"What were you doing in the woods?" Henry asked. "What was *she* doing in the woods?"

"Drawing. We were both drawing."

The Aldens were silent for several minutes. Then Henry said, "Grandfather, there was a big broken window in town on Fifth Street. The store that used to be Gerry's General Store."

"I heard about that," Mr. Alden said. "I was in town about an hour ago, getting my hair cut, when Mrs. Leob reported the broken window. The police think it was vandalism."

"What's vandalism?" Benny asked.

"That means someone broke the window on purpose," Henry said. "Why do the police think it was vandalism?"

"Because just inside the broken window, on the floor, were several golf balls."

"Golf balls!" Jessie exclaimed. She and Henry looked at each other.

"Very curious," Henry said.

"What's curious about that?" Benny asked.

Jessie told the family about what had happened at practice, how Danielle tripped Kayla with a golf ball, and how Kayla put the ball in her pocket and carried it home.

"That is funny!" Benny said. "Usually you never hear anything about golf balls! But suddenly there are golf balls everywhere!"

"There may be something about the broken window in the evening paper," Henry said. "Grandfather, may I get your newspaper?"

"Certainly," Mr. Alden said.

Mr. Alden's newspaper was still folded just inside the front door. Henry picked up the newspaper and returned to the table. He rolled off the rubber band and opened the paper. There, on the Town News page, was a short mention of the broken window, only a few sentences in length. Henry read the sentences to his family:

"The window of Gerry's General Store was found broken this afternoon. Golf balls were found on the floor, just inside. The police suspect vandalism."

"We didn't learn anything at all new from that," Jessie said.

"Except now we have another mystery to solve!" Benny said.

CHAPTER 7

The Mystery of the Golf Balls

"Did you hear?" Danielle said to Jessie the next day on the black-top.

The paved area in back of the school where the kids waited for the bell was called the black-top because the pavement was so dark. The only problem with waiting on the black-top was the asphalt heated up on hot days. It was still early, and already Jessie could feel the heat coming up from the pavement. On hot days, the black-top smelled of tar.

"Hear what?" Jessie asked.

"Kayla broke the window of the old General Store," Danielle said.

Jessie was so startled, all she could say was, "What?!"

"A golf ball was found just inside the window. Remember when Kayla left practice? She was mad. And she had a golf ball in her pocket."

"She did not break the window," Jessie said. "She couldn't have. Henry and I saw her with the golf ball after the window was already broken."

"Who else would have done it?" Danielle said. "Don't you remember how mad she was?"

"I remember," Jessie said. "She was mad because *you* tripped her!"

"She wasn't just mad at me," Danielle said to Jessie. "She was angry in general because now she doesn't get to be mascot."

"We don't know that for sure," Jessie said. "Someone wrote a letter and there is an investigation."

"I don't think she will be allowed to be

mascot," Danielle said. "I don't think Coach Olson likes Kayla very much. I don't think he likes Kayla's mother, either. She is very pushy."

"Listen," Jessie said. "Kayla couldn't have broken the window. I saw Kayla with that golf ball after the window was broken. Besides, the newspaper said several golf balls were found in the store. Kayla only had one."

Danielle shrugged. "The newspaper could have accidentally printed 'golf balls,' when they meant 'golf ball.'"

"I really doubt that," Jessie said.

Ashley was standing nearby with a group of girls. "Hey, Ashley!" Danielle called. "Don't you think Kayla was the one who broke the window?"

"You're spreading rumors!" Jessie said to Danielle.

Danielle ignored Jessie and said, "Hey, Ashley, what do you think? Kayla was the one with a golf ball, right?"

Ashley gave a quick shrug, but didn't look directly at either Jessie or Danielle. "Could be," Ashley said. "She was awfully mad at you." Ashley turned away.

Jessie watched Ashley curiously. There was something strange about the way Ashley acted.

***

"I did *not* break that window," Kayla said adamantly when someone asked her about it during lunch. Jessie was eating her lunch with a few friends at the next table. She hadn't noticed that Kayla had been sitting not far away, eating her lunch alone.

"Who else would have done it?" the girl asked.

"I don't know!" Kayla said. Ordinarily Kayla was aloof and a bit detached. Now there was deep passion in her voice.

Jessie felt she had to do something. She excused herself from her friends, and walked to Kayla's table.

"I know Kayla didn't do it," Jessie said.

"How do you know?" asked a boy sitting nearby.

"My brother Henry and I saw Kayla walking home yesterday. She still had the golf ball in her pocket. At the same time, we saw the window already broken. Besides, the police report said there were golf balls found inside the window. Kayla had only one."

Kayla looked at Jessie with gratitude and astonishment. The other kids were silent.

"So I know Kayla didn't do it," Jessie said quietly.

"Who do you think did it, then?" another boy sitting nearby asked Jessie.

"I don't know," Jessie said. "But not Kayla."

"Maybe," suggested one of Jessie's friends, who had come over to listen better, "whoever wrote the letter also broke the window because they want to make Kayla look bad."

"That's what my parents think," Kayla said. "They think someone did it and is blaming it on me." Kayla looked directly at Ashley and Danielle. Once again Ashley got a strange look on her face. She turned red and looked away.

Yes, there was something very odd in Ashley's behavior.

***

Jessie's gym period was the last period of the day. Ordinarily she liked having gym class last. She played hard at sports, which meant after gym she was tired and ready for a very long rest. In a heat wave like this one, though, it meant gym class was during the hottest time of the day.

Jessie's class was playing soccer. Soccer was a fall sport, so the first unit of the school year was always soccer. Because so many people liked soccer, Coach Olson joked that playing soccer first was a good way to get everyone excited about returning to school.

Coach Olson watched the class play. He held a clipboard and made notes. After the game, he met with each girl for a few moments and gave pointers to help them improve.

When it was Jessie's turn, he said, "I'm pleased with your game. Your dribbling and ball control are particularly good. You need to work on keeping an eye on the whole field so you know where there is an open player."

Jessie understood exactly what he meant. Sometimes she was so busy watching the ball, she forgot to keep an eye on the entire field to keep track of where the players were. It was particularly important for her to keep an eye on the entire field because she was team captain.

Then Coach Olson startled her by saying, "Jessie, I believe you are the girl who should be an international mascot. You're a true team player. You are a credit to the game. Mia thinks so, too."

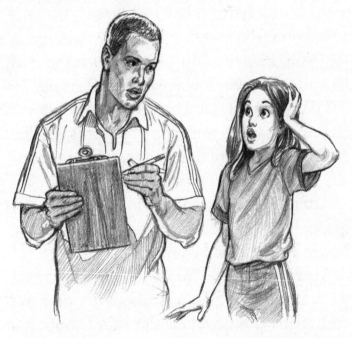

"I would love to be the mascot," Jessie said. "Don't get me wrong. Going to Brazil! Watching an international tournament! It would all be thrilling. But—" Jessie broke off and looked away. This was the hard part to explain. "I just wouldn't feel right about taking the honor away from Kayla because of an anonymous letter."

"If Kayla doesn't deserve it," the coach said, "but you do, you're not really taking anything away from her."

"I know Kayla didn't break the window. I told you. Henry and I saw her with the golf ball after the window was already broken."

"We will find out who broke the window," the coach said. "Don't worry about that. The police have ways of figuring these things out."

***

After school that day, Violet went to the glade in the woods to draw. She secretly hoped Kayla would come again.

After filling two pages of her sketchpad with drawings, she was about to give up and return home when she heard footsteps coming down the trail. Sure enough, Kayla emerged from the path carrying a sketch pad and a beach blanket.

Violet smiled. Without a word, Kayla spread her blanket near Violet and took out her drawing pencils. The girls drew in silence for a long time. At last, Violet said, "You should sign up for the after school art program. We meet on Mondays and get drawing and painting lessons."

"I would like to," Kayla said. "But I don't think my parents would like that."

"Why not?"

"This is soccer season. They want me to practice. My sister got on the high school soccer team. They want me to be able to make the high school team, too."

"But you will!" Violet said. "You're so good!"

"A good player can always get better," Kayla said. "That's what my parents say."

What startled Violet most was there was sadness in Kayla's voice.

"You don't want to practice soccer?" Violet asked.

"Not all the time," Kayla said.

"Why did you want to be a mascot?"

"I didn't. My parents filled out the application for me. I didn't even know they had done that."

The two girls went back to their drawings. After a while, Kayla said, "My parents have high hopes for me. Mom says I'm a natural. Dad says I have real talent for soccer. They think I can be the best soccer player in the family, if I apply myself."

"But you don't want to," Violet said, deeply astonished. Kayla wasn't at all the kind of person people thought she was.

"I used to think all children played soccer," Kayla said. "I used to think all families spent their weekends playing soccer or watching soccer. I was in third grade before I realized not all families are like mine."

"Most people would think you're lucky," Violet said, "to have parents who play soccer with you all the time."

"I know," Kayla said. That was all she said. Violet, who understood how it felt to be inward and shy, didn't push her to say any more.

CHAPTER 8

The Clue of the Broken Glass

Benny was at the kitchen table doing homework when Mrs. McGregor called out to Grandfather, "Would you like some iced coffee before dinner?"

"I would love some!" he responded. "Thanks!"

Benny was adding a row of numbers. He was concentrating so hard he hardly noticed the grinding of the coffeemaker, or even the sound of Mrs. McGregor whistling as she worked.

Suddenly Mrs. McGregor let out a little shriek, then exclaimed, "Oh, no!"

Benny, startled, dropped his pencil. "What's the matter?"

"Oh, fiddlesticks!" she said. "Would you look at that! The glass broke. I put ice into the coffee, and bang! The glass broke!"

"How?"

"It was silly of me. The glass was too thin, and got too hot. Then I put in the ice. Oh fiddlesticks!"

Sure enough, there on the counter, were pieces of broken glass.

"I'll help clean it up!" Benny shouted.

"No, please stay back. I don't want you to get cut. Stay here. I'll get the dustpan."

Just then the phone rang. "Stay put," Mrs. McGregor said. "Let your grandfather answer it. There might be glass on the floor. I don't want you to step on it."

Benny heard grandfather's steps in the hallway. "Hello," Grandfather said. There were a few moments of silence while Grandfather listened to whoever was talking.

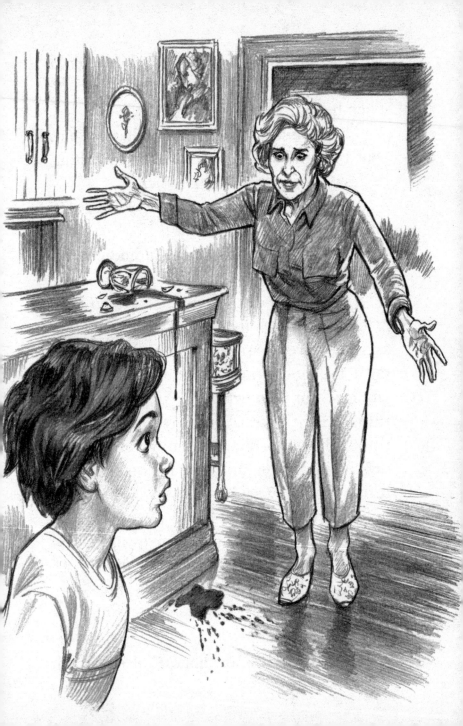

Then he said: "Really? Jessie?"

"That is quite an honor," Grandfather said, "but I am not sure how Jessie will feel about it. Yes . . . yes. . .I will talk to her."

"All right, then," he said. "Goodbye." He hung up the phone.

Jessie came into the room. "Grandfather?" she asked. "What is it?"

"That was Coach Olson," Mr. Alden said. "He is still working on the investigation. He says the investigation will not be complete until the police figure out who broke the window, but meanwhile, he believes all the things in the letter about Kayla are true. He thinks the honor should go to Jessie, who he says is much nicer and more nurturing of her teammates. So what he wants to do, when the police figure out who broke the window, is suggest to the committee that Jessie should be invited to Brazil as a child mascot instead."

Jessie and Benny looked at each other.

"I told him it was an honor," Grandfather said quietly.

"Of course it's an honor!" Jessie said,

recovering from her surprise enough to speak. "Going to Brazil to see the international tournament would be amazing! But I can't possibly go! I just don't think it's fair to Kayla! This will be so humiliating for Kayla. It's wrong to give it to me instead."

"Coach Olson doesn't think so," Grandfather said. "He said the committee wants the mascot to be someone who sets a good example for the sport, not just plays well."

"It just isn't right," Jessie said.

"If that's how you feel," Grandfather said, "We can tell Coach Olson not to nominate you because you don't want to accept."

"I'll think about it," Jessie said.

***

After the children finished their homework, Jessie called a meeting so they could look at their clues.

"We have to get to the bottom of this," she said. "I will not be able to accept the invitation to be mascot as long as it looks like someone has it in for Kayla."

"People are wrong about Kayla," Violet said. "Kayla is a nice person. I know she is. People just don't understand her. I don't think she cares that much about soccer. I think she only plays because her parents want her to."

"I will tell you what I'm wondering," Henry said. "I am starting to wonder if Coach Olson is behind this. It's clear Kayla's mother and Coach Olson don't like each other much. It's also clear Coach Olson doesn't like Kayla. And Jessie is his favorite. I've heard kids say that."

"You think Coach Olson wrote the letter?" Jessie asked. "I can't believe a coach would do that. Anyway, why would he write an anonymous letter? Why wouldn't he just call the committee and say Kayla should not be mascot because she sets a bad example?"

"Maybe because he doesn't want Kayla's family any madder at him," Henry said.

"But why would Coach Olson write a letter from the library computer?" Jessie asked. "Wouldn't he know about the automatic save function?"

"Maybe he wants people to think a kid did it," Henry said.

"I just can't believe it was Coach Olson," Jessie said. "I think it was one of the girls on the red team. Maybe Ashley or Danielle or someone who is staying quiet."

"What about that broken window?" Benny said. "Probably the same person who wrote the letter also broke the window so Kayla would be blamed, right?"

"It sort of looks like that," Henry said.

"Coach Olson would never break a window," Jessie said.

"I agree with that," Henry said. "So maybe it wasn't Coach Olson after all."

"We need to figure out who broke the window!" Benny said. "Then we might have a clue who wrote the letter!"

The others nodded in agreement.

"We don't have any real clues at all about the broken window," Henry said. "Do we?"

"None," Jessie said. "Maybe fewer clues than who wrote the letter."

"What do we know about the window?"

Henry asked. "Was there anything at all unusual?"

They were all silent. "The only thing I can think of," Jessie said, "is when we went to look at the broken window, the air conditioner was blowing. I guess that means someone was inside and turned it on."

"Also it was a very old window," Henry said. "The wood was splintered and the glass was a murky color."

Suddenly Benny said, "Maybe it's like putting ice in hot coffee!"

The others looked at Benny, puzzled.

Seeing their expressions, Benny said, "Putting ice in hot coffee can break glass if the glass is too thin! Just ask Mrs. MacGregor!"

The children went to find Mrs. MacGregor, who said, "Yes, indeed. That was silly of me. The ice in the hot coffee broke the glass. I should have known that glass was too thin."

"I wonder if the same thing can happen with windows," Henry said. "Remember Beck said something about having to be careful with these old windows in the summer."

"After dinner," Jessie said, "let's go ask him."

***

After dinner all four children walked the five blocks to Mr. Beck's house. He lived in the part of town where the houses were mostly painted white, with clapboard sides and picket fences in front. The lawns and flower beds were neatly trimmed. Mr. Beck's white van was parked in his driveway. *Beck Handyman Service* was printed in red and blue letters.

"Looks like he's here," Jessie said.

"I want to ring the doorbell!" Benny shouted. He liked ringing doorbells.

"If you keep shouting like that," Violet said, smiling, "we won't have to ring the doorbell!"

Benny ran to the door and rang the doorbell. He rang it a second time. He was about to ring the bell a third time when Jessie ran and caught his hand and said, "Benny! That's enough!"

Mr. Beck opened the door and smiled at the children. "Look who's here! All four Alden children! What can I do for you?"

"We have a question," Henry said. "On Saturday when you were working at our house, you said you have to watch out with these old windows in the summer. What did you mean?"

"The windows in your house were getting tight and hard to open," he said. "Old windows are fragile and can break easily."

"What would you think if an air conditioner was running on a very hot day," Henry said, "so the air inside was very cold...could that make a window break?"

"Extreme temperature changes are very bad for old glass," Mr. Beck said. "Very cold inside, and very hot outside? Yes, that could cause a spontaneous break. Why?"

"Spontaneous!" Benny cried. "Like putting ice in hot coffee! The glass can break!"

"Exactly," said Mr. Beck.

"The air conditioning was running in the old Gerry's General Store building," Henry said. "The police think it was vandalism. People are blaming Kayla. But maybe the old window broke because of the cold inside and hot outside."

"I read about that broken window in the newspaper," Mr. Beck said. "The newspaper didn't say anything about an air conditioner running."

"The air conditioner was definitely running," Jessie said. "I'm surprised Mrs. Leob didn't mention that to the police. I wonder why it was on."

"That was an old building," said Mr. Beck. "The air conditioner was probably old, too. It probably just went haywire. Turned on by itself. The windows got icy cold, the sun beat down, and *wham*, the window broke."

"Perhaps we should tell the police," Violet said. "They might not know the inside was freezing and that extreme temperature changes can cause old glass to break."

"I will do that," Mr. Beck said. "I will head over there right away. They can investigate to see if that was what broke the window."

The children thanked Mr. Beck. They all said goodbye.

When the children were back on the sidewalk heading home, Jessie said, "It's nice to know the broken window probably wasn't vandalism. The problem is, we're no closer to figuring out who wrote that letter and caused Kayla all these problems."

Violet said, "At least people will stop blaming Kayla for the broken window."

"I was really starting to think Ashley had broken the window," Jessie said. "She kept acting strangely about the golf ball."

"Maybe there is still a clue there," Henry said. "There was something strange about all those golf balls on the floor of the store. Why don't you just ask her what she knows about the golf ball? You're the team captain, after all. The ball was used to trip a team member. You have a good reason to ask her."

"All right, I'll ask her tomorrow," Jessie said. "Maybe there still is a connection between the golf balls and the letter writer, even though I can't imagine what the connection can possibly be."

***

That night, long after the rest of the family was asleep, Violet heard Jessie tossing in her bed.

"Are you awake?" Violet whispered.

"Yes," Jessie said. "I'm thinking about Kayla. Why are you awake?"

"I keep thinking about Kayla, too," Violet said.

The only light in the room came from a small night light in the bathroom just down the hallway. There was just enough light so Violet could see the outline of her stuffed animals on the shelf near her bed.

"I would love to be an international soccer mascot," Jessie whispered. "But not like this. Not because someone else is having bad fortune."

"I know what you mean," Violet whispered back.

"If we don't get to the bottom of this," Jessie said, "I'll have to say I don't want to go."

Just then, words popped into Violet's head: *Things aren't always as they seem.*

Violet's teacher had said that once. Violet agreed completely that things were not always as they seemed. For example, a lot of people disliked Kayla. A lot of people were jealous of Kayla, too. So it seemed like someone who didn't like her and was jealous of her wrote the mean letter. *But maybe that wasn't what happened at all*, Violet realized.

She thought about the golf balls. Because golf balls were found inside Gerry's General Store, and because Kayla had a golf ball in her hand, so it seemed like there was a connection between Kayla and the broken window. But what if there was more to the story?

Violet knew that sometimes, with mysteries, the clue is where something doesn't quite feel right.

For Violet, the part that didn't feel right was Kayla's attitude toward soccer. She didn't seem to even like soccer. Who would have thought that?

Everyone criticized Kayla for not being a team player. But if she didn't even like soccer, no wonder she wasn't a good team player.

Violet put her head on the pillow and closed her eyes. Jessie's breathing was so deep and steady, Violet knew she had fallen asleep. Violet still felt puzzled, but she felt comforted as always by the nearness of her sister. Soon she, too, fell asleep.

CHAPTER 9

A Confession

The next morning, at school, lots of Jessie's classmates came to congratulate her on being asked to be mascot.

Jessie said thank you, always adding, "But I don't think I'll go. I don't think it's fair to Kayla."

"I'm *sure* you'll go, Jessie," Danielle said coldly.

Jessie turned to look at Danielle, astonished.

"Everyone keeps thinking I wrote that letter," Danielle said, "because I don't like

Kayla. Here's what I wonder. I wonder if *Jessie* wrote the letter because she knew Coach Olson likes her best, so she knew she'd get to go to Brazil as mascot!"

"I did not write that letter," Jessie said, horrified.

Just then, Ashley walked over to join them. "Maybe it was Jessie who wrote the letter!" Ashley said.

Jessie folded her arms across her chest and looked at Ashley. "Tell me about that golf ball Danielle used to trip Kayla," Jessie said. "What do you know about it?"

As before, the mention of the golf ball had a strange effect on Ashley. She looked quickly away and didn't say anything. She rocked on the balls of her feet, as if she wanted to run away.

No doubt, there was something going on with Ashley and that golf ball.

"It's okay," Jessie said gently. "You can tell me. I don't think you broke the window. Something seems strange, though, about the whole thing. A bunch of golf balls were found inside the store. Danielle used a golf ball to trip Kayla. Then people started blaming Kayla for breaking the window when I know she didn't."

Ashley had a pained, guilty look on her face. Jessie suspected Ashley was about to make a confession. She was thus surprised when Ashley cried, "I didn't break the window either! I promise."

"I know you didn't," Jessie said. "Mr. Beck, the handyman, knows about old windows. He said it probably broke by itself."

"Well, good, because I didn't break the window," Ashley said.

"Then why do you act strangely every time someone mentions the golf ball?" Jessie asked.

Ashley narrowed her eyes. A moment passed. Then another. Jessie thought Ashley was about to say something mean. Instead, she said, "I was walking to practice on Wednesday, and I went by the old store. The window was broken and inside were some golf balls. I reached in and picked one up. While we were waiting for practice, Danielle and I were rolling it back and forth."

"I see," Jessie said. "The truth is that you stole the golf ball."

Ashley looked horrified. "It was just laying there! It didn't belong to anyone! The store was abandoned! It really wasn't stealing!"

Jessie didn't answer.

"It wasn't," Ashley said. Then she softened and looked genuinely frightened. "Was it?"

"It *was* stealing," Jessie said. "Why did you take it?"

"It was just sitting there inside the window. I don't know. I shouldn't have."

"Just go put it back," Jessie said.

"I would, but Kayla still has it. I can't ask her for it back. She'll wonder why I'm asking. Then she'll figure out I stole it, then she'll tell everyone I stole it to get back at me for being mean."

"Maybe she won't," Jessie said. Then she had an idea. "Do you want me to get it back from her?"

"Would you?" Ashley said. "Oh, thank you!"

***

Jessie was walking home from school when she was surprised by a tap on her shoulder.

She turned. There was Kayla, smiling. "Thanks," Kayla said.

Jessie knew right away Kayla was thanking her for standing up for her about the window.

"It was nothing," Jessie said. "I just knew you didn't break that window."

"It was awfully nice of you," Kayla said.

Then Jessie remembered Ashley and the golf ball. "Oh, by the way, do you still have that golf ball?"

"Yes," Kayla said. "Why?"

"I know who it belongs to. Will you give it to me so I can return it?"

"Sure!" Kayla waved, then walked off in the direction of her own house.

***

When Jessie arrived home, she immediately went to look for Henry. He was already in his bedroom, sitting at his desk, doing homework. When she entered his room, he set down his pencil and turned to her. She told him everything, including the mean thing Danielle had suggested.

"Someone in my class said that, too," Henry said. "Someone who doesn't know you at all suggested you wrote the letter so you could be mascot."

Jessie sat down gloomily. "We have to figure out who wrote the letter!" she said.

Henry said, "Let's gather everyone together so we can go over our clues. It's snack time, anyway."

All four children sat together at the table in the kitchen eating their after-school snack. Mrs. McGregor had made banana bread, which they ate with milk. "This is the best banana bread Mrs. McGregor has ever made!" Benny said, as he helped himself to another slice.

The children went over all their clues. Given how many people disliked Kayla, they were surprised to realize they had only three real suspects: Mr. Olson, Danielle, and Ashley. Jessie added another name. "Mia said she thought I should be mascot, so she is a suspect, too."

"Who's Mia?" Benny asked.

"She's the high school girl who helps coaches my team," Jessie said.

The problem was Jessie was pretty sure neither Danielle or Ashley had written the letter. Nobody really believed Mr. Olson had done it. And there wasn't much to connect Mia to the letter, either.

The Alden children looked at each other in silence.

Suddenly Violet said, "There is one other suspect we haven't thought of who might have written that letter."

Everyone looked at her.

"Who?" Henry asked.

"Kayla," Violet said.

The children looked at her, stunned.

"She doesn't even like soccer," Violet said. "She told me. Her parents filled out the application. I think they push her to play soccer when she'd rather not. I think she'd rather draw."

"That explains why she hasn't acted upset about not being mascot," Jessie said.

"Do you think she sabotaged her own chances?" Henry asked. "Why not just say she didn't want to be mascot?"

"Maybe she thought the letter would be easier than telling her parents the truth," Violet said.

The children were quiet, considering this.

"Well," Jessie said. "Her mother is very forceful."

Henry said, "Kayla's new in town, so she might not know about the automatic save function at the library."

"Even if she knew," Jessie said, "why would she care? Nobody would suspect her. They'd think it was Danielle or someone else who is mean to her."

"If Kayla wrote the letter," Henry said, "she'll never tell anyone."

"She might tell me," Violet said.

"How are you going to get her to tell you?" Jessie asked.

"I don't know yet," Violet said.

***

Kayla was in the glade with her sketch pad

when Violet arrived. Violet smiled, sat down, and took out her pencils. To Violet's surprise, she also took out a golf ball.

"Can you give this to Jessie for me?"

"Certainly," Violet said. They drew for a long time in silence. At last, Violet put her pencil down and said, "There is something bad happening. It has to do with Jessie."

"Jessie?" Kayla looked instantly concerned.

"People are saying Jessie wrote that letter to the mascot committee because she wanted to be mascot. People say she knew she was Coach Olson's favorite and if your chances were ruined, she'd get to be mascot."

"Everyone should know Jessie would never do something like that," Kayla said.

Kayla frowned and went back to her sketch pad. The two girls drew for a while in silence. Violet was not concentrating on her drawing. She sensed that Kayla wasn't either.

Violet took a deep breath and said, "Do you know what I think?" Violet knew it was easier for shy people to listen to other people's ideas than to answer direct questions. So she said,

"I think you wrote the letter." She said this in a matter-of-fact way.

"Ridiculous," Kayla said. She went on drawing.

"I just thought maybe you wrote the letter because your parents are so serious about soccer."

"They are serious," Kayla said. "*Too* serious, if you ask me."

They drew in silence again. After a while, Kayla said, "Do people really think Jessie would write that letter?"

"It looks bad, doesn't it? Someone writes a letter, then Jessie gets to be mascot. You can see how people might think that."

Kayla sprang to her feet. "Well it's not true! Jessie did *not* write the letter." Kayla scooped up her pencils and sketchpad. "I have to go now," she said, and ran off through the woods.

Violet scooped up her own pencils and sketchpad and ran after her. Kayla was a good runner, much better than Violet. Violet had to run her fastest to keep up. When Kayla

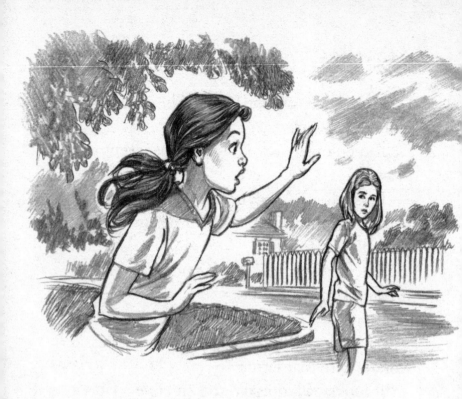

turned right at the street, Violet understood
Kayla was heading toward the soccer field.

***

Jessie had come early to soccer practice
that day. Coach Olson, and a few of the girls,
were already there. Mia had said she couldn't
coach, so Coach Olson said he'd be there too
so Henry wouldn't be on his own.

Jessie waved to Coach Olson. He waved
back. She walked purposely toward him.

"Hey, Jessie, what's up?" he asked.

"I've been thinking," she said. "I believe someone is sabotaging Kayla. I just don't feel right accepting the invitation to be mascot because—"

They both looked up to see Mrs. Thompson marching across the street toward them.

"Oh, no," Coach Olson said. "It looks like something else has happened."

"Has anyone seen Kayla?" Mrs. Thompson asked loudly.

Coach Olson looked around. "She doesn't seem to be here yet."

"I haven't been able to find her all afternoon. Lately she's been disappearing for hours at a time."

"Here she comes now!" Jessie said, pointing.

Kayla jogged toward them. Tucked under her arm was a sketch pad. Her face was flushed from the heat, her neck and forehead wet with perspiration.

That was when Jessie noticed that Violet, too, was running from the same direction. Violet was panting. Jessie ran for her own water bottle and gave it to Violet, who drank some, then splashed water on her face.

"Whew!" Violet said. "It's hot!"

"What's going on?" Jessie whispered.

"I'm not completely sure," Violet whispered back.

"Where have you been?" Mrs. Thompson asked Kayla.

"In the woods, drawing." Kayla's voice was low and remarkably steady for someone who had just sprinted in the heat.

"Why?" Mrs. Thompson asked.

Instead of answering the question, Kayla said, "I cannot have people saying that Jessie wrote that letter sabotaging me. Jessie is much too nice. She didn't do it."

"And how do you know that?" Mrs. Thompson said.

"Because *I* wrote the letter," Kayla said.

There was stunned silence. Then Mrs. Thompson said, "What?"

"I never thought it would blow up this way!" Kayla said. "I never thought there would be a big scandal. I thought you'd keep it all hush-hush. I thought you'd be embarrassed. I didn't think you'd march onto the soccer field and tell the whole town about it!"

Mrs. Thompson stared, astonished. She opened her mouth to speak, but then closed her mouth. There was a long silence. Jessie found herself smiling. She supposed Mrs. Thompson wasn't often at a loss for words.

At last, Mrs. Thompson asked, "Why on earth would you do such a thing?"

Kayla didn't answer.

Violet leaned and whispered to Jessie, "She wrote the letter because she didn't want to play soccer anymore."

Jessie stepped forward and, to Mrs. Thompson, said, "Ma'am, maybe Kayla wrote the letter because she didn't want to play soccer any more. Maybe she didn't want to be a mascot."

"Oh, don't be silly," Mrs. Thompson snapped.

"Well, I didn't!" Kayla said. "It was too much! Soccer, soccer, soccer. All the time. Every day. Nothing else but soccer! I told you I wanted to do the drawing class and you said, 'but what about soccer.'"

Violet squeezed Jessie's hand.

Things are not what they seem.

Kayla wasn't a snooty show-off, like everyone thought. She was unhappy. She was shy and quiet. She wanted to be left in peace, with her sketch pad. She acted badly because she didn't want to play any more.

Kayla turned to Jessie. "I hope you decide to accept the invitation. You deserve it. You'd be a wonderful mascot."

CHAPTER 10

Prime Time Soccer

Thousands of people cheered and waved flags and banners. The stadium was so crowded, the Aldens held on to each other as they made their way to their seats. All around people were speaking different languages.

"I can't believe we are in Rio de Janeiro!" Henry said.

"I'll bet there are one million people in this stadium!" Benny said.

"Almost," Henry said. "This stadium holds almost seventy-five thousand people."

"Seventy-five thousand!" Benny repeated, astonished. "How many zeroes is that?"

"Three," said Henry.

Up ahead, a child accidentally dropped the churro he was eating. Benny watched the churro drop and said, "Poor Watch. He'd love to be here!"

"He could make all the noise he wanted," Violet said. "And nobody would even hear."

"And he could eat the food people are dropping," Benny said.

Benny liked the smells of all the different foods. Most of the food for sale in the booths he didn't recognize, but they all smelled delicious. He looked forward to lunch! No boring hot dogs and peanuts for him! He was looking forward to trying new Brazilian food.

Aloud he said, "This is much better than a coupon for a free cone at Igloo Ice Cream! A million times better!"

Grandfather, Henry, Violet, and Benny sat in the special seats reserved for family members of mascots.

"The opening ceremony will start soon," Henry said, checking his watch.

"Yay!" Benny shouted.

Violet smiled. She was happy things worked out so well. Somewhere in these thousands of people, Kayla was here with her parents. Kayla's parents still wanted to come to the tournament. Kayla was happy to go, as long as she didn't have to walk onto the field in front of millions of people and as long as she didn't have to play soccer if she didn't want to. The Thompsons were staying at the same hotel as the Aldens. That morning, they'd all had breakfast together.

Kayla's parents let her sign up for the Monday after school art class. Kayla was multi-talented. She was a good artist and a good soccer player. She also knew how to be a good friend.

Ashley's attitude toward Kayla changed as well. After Jessie gave her the golf ball, and Ashley returned it to the store, Ashley stopped being mean to Kayla. In fact, the next time Danielle started saying something unkind to Kayla, Ashley stopped her.

The marching band came onto the field, but the crowd was cheering so loudly the children could only hear the beating of the drums. Then came the spectacular fireworks.

"Look at that one over there!" Benny shouted, pointing to the sky. "Fireworks!"

"I like that one!" Violet shouted, pointing. "Lavender fireworks! Amazing!"

A singer stood on the stage and sang. The crowd quieted so the children could hear her singing. Her voice was smooth and rich. Violet could not understand the words, but the music was breathtakingly beautiful.

Next, two expert soccer players did a demonstration. They dribbled the ball up and down the field, showing the most amazing footwork—kicking the ball in surprising directions, kicking it into the air and bouncing it up and down on their heads and shoulders, keeping it moving in the air without ever using their hands.

"They're so good," Violet said, "they make Kayla look like a beginner!"

"I wish I could do that!" Benny said.

"Maybe you can," Grandfather suggested. "If you practice enough."

"I am going to practice as soon as we get home!" Benny said. "I am going to practice and practice! Maybe one day I will be in a real tournament!"

At last, it was time for the child mascots to walk onto the field with the players. The Aldens watched excitedly for Jessie.

"There she is!" Benny shouted. "I see her!"

Indeed, Jessie was just then walking on the field alongside one of the team members. The spectators cheered and stamped their feet. People waved streamers. Jessie turned and waved.

Henry, Benny, and even Violet clapped loudly, stamped their feet, and shouted, "Yay, Jessie! Yay, Jessie!"

Benny bounded out of his seat, pointed to the field, and shouted at the top of his voice, "That's my sister over there." He jumped up and down a few times. "That's my sister over there!"

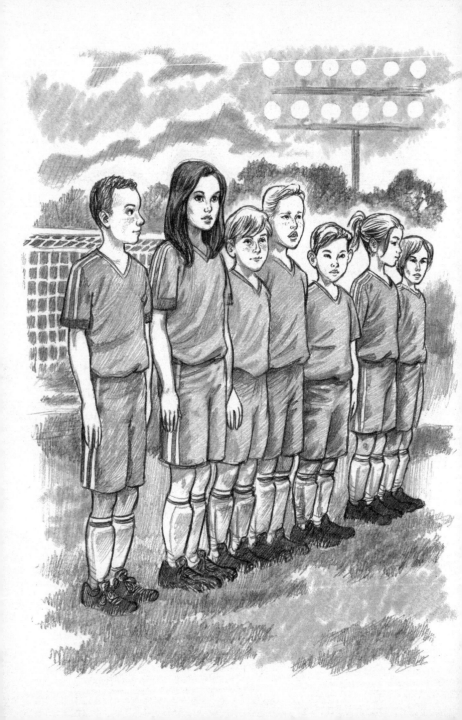

Jessie had, by now, walked all the way around the field. Just before she stepped out of the spotlight, she turned once more and waved to her family.

Grandfather smiled. "I am so proud of her. I am proud of all of you."

THE BOXCAR CHILDREN BEGINNING

by Patricia MacLachlan

Before they were the Boxcar Children, Henry, Jessie, Violet, and Benny Alden lived with their parents on Fair Meadow Farm.

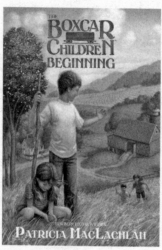

978-0-8075-6617-6
US $5.99 paperback

Although times are hard, they're happy—"the best family of all," Mama likes to say. And when a traveling family needs shelter from a winter storm, the Aldens help, and make new friends. But the spring and summer bring events that will change all their lives forever.

Newbery Award-winning author Patricia MacLachlan tells a wonderfully moving story of the Alden children's origins.

* * *

"Fans will enjoy this picture of life 'before.'"—*Publishers Weekly*

"An approachable lead-in that serves to fill in the background both for confirmed fans and readers new to the series." —*Kirkus Reviews*

THE BOXCAR CHILDREN SPOOKTACULAR SPECIAL

created by Gertrude Chandler Warner

Three spooky stories in one big book!

From ghosts to zombies to a haunting in their very own backyard, the Boxcar Children have plenty of spooktacular adventures in these three exciting mysteries.

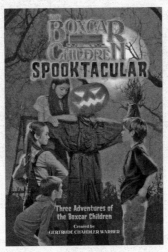

978-0-8075-7605-2
US $9.99 paperback

THE ZOMBIE PROJECT
The story about the Winding River zombie is just an old legend. But Benny sees a strange figure lurching through the woods and thinks the zombie could be real!

THE MYSTERY OF THE HAUNTED BOXCAR
One night the Aldens see a mysterious light shining inside the boxcar where they once lived. Soon they discover spooky new clues to the old train car's past!

THE PUMPKIN HEAD MYSTERY
Every year the Aldens help out with the fun at a pumpkin farm. Can they find out why a ghost with a jack-o'-lantern head is haunting the hayrides?

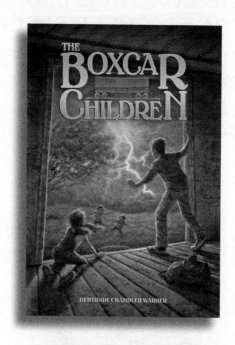

#1 THE BOXCAR CHILDREN
THE BOXCAR CHILDREN® MYSTERIES
HC 978-0-8075-0851-0
$15.99/$17.99 Canada
PB 978-0-8075-0852-7
$5.99/$6.99 Canada
"One warm night four children stood in front of a bakery. No one knew them. No one knew where they had come from." So begins Gertrude Chandler Warner's beloved story about four orphans who run away and find shelter in an abandoned boxcar. There they manage to live all on their own, and at last, find love and security from an unexpected source.

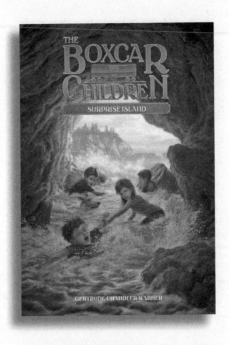

#2 SURPRISE ISLAND
THE BOXCAR CHILDREN® MYSTERIES
HC 978-0-8075-7673-1
$15.99/$17.99 Canada
PB 978-0-8075-7674-8
$5.99/$6.99 Canada
The Boxcar Children have a home with their
grandfather now—but their adventures are just
beginning! Their first adventure is to spend the
summer camping on their own private island.
The island is full of surprises, including a kind
stranger with a secret.

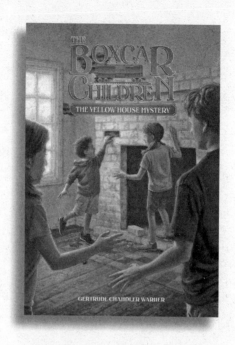

#3 THE YELLOW HOUSE MYSTERY
THE BOXCAR CHILDREN® MYSTERIES

HC 978-0-8075-9365-3
$15.99/$17.99 Canada
PB 978-0-8075-9366-0
$5.99/$6.99 Canada
Henry, Jessie, Violet, and Benny Alden discover
that a mystery surrounds the rundown yellow
house on Surprise Island. The children find a
letter and other clues that lead them to the trail
of a man who vanished from the house.

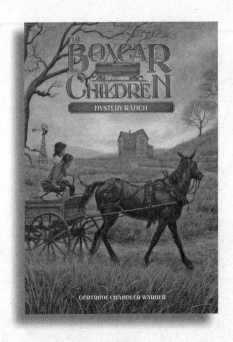

#4 MYSTERY RANCH
THE BOXCAR CHILDREN® MYSTERIES
HC 978-0-8075-5390-9
$15.99/$17.99 Canada
PB 978-0-8075-5391-6
$5.99/$6.99 Canada
Henry, Jessie, Violet, and Benny Alden just
found out they have an Aunt Jane and travel out
west to spend the summer on her ranch. While
there, they make an amazing discovery about
the ranch that will change Aunt Jane's life.

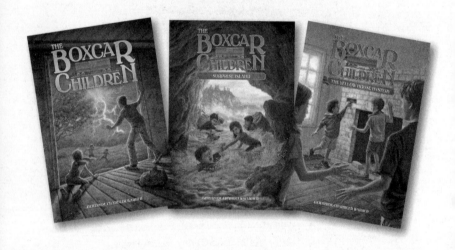

GERTRUDE CHANDLER WARNER discovered when she was teaching that many readers who like an exciting story could find no books that were both easy and fun to read. She decided to try to meet this need, and her first book, *The Boxcar Children*, quickly proved she had succeeded.

Miss Warner drew on her own experiences to write the mystery. As a child she spent hours watching trains go by on the tracks opposite her family home. She often dreamed about what it would be like to set up housekeeping in a caboose or freight car—the situation the Alden children find themselves in.

While the mystery element is central to each of Miss Warner's books, she never thought of them as strictly juvenile mysteries. She liked to stress the Aldens' independence and resourcefulness and their solid New England devotion to using up and making do. The Aldens go about most of their adventures with as little adult supervision as possible—something else that delights young readers.

Miss Warner lived in Putnam, Connecticut, until her death in 1979. During her lifetime, she received hundreds of letters from girls and boys telling her how much they liked her books.